THE
WELLNESS
FOR LIFE
WORKBOOK

PHYSICAL ACTIVITY • NUTRITION • WEIGHT CONTROL
STRESS MANAGEMENT • CHEMICAL INDEPENDENCE

Thomas A. Murphy

and

Dianne Murphy

FITNESS PUBLICATIONS

First edition (The Personal Fitness Workbook) 1982
Second edition 1983
Third edition (Wellness For Life) 1984

FITNESS PUBLICATIONS
San Diego, California

ISBN 0-9611482-2-5

This workbook
is dedicated to the activation of your capacity
to enjoy wellness for life . . . .

TABLE OF CONTENTS

INTRODUCTION

Over time, you are either strengthened or weakened by what you do with yourself on a regular basis. Your present state of wellness and your life-long well-being are largely determined by your accustomed patterns of thought and behavior. The way you eat, your level of physical activity, how you handle stress and your avoidance of chemical dependencies all affect your ability to function effectively and to enthusiastically partake of the good life. To a large extent, these aspects of your lifestyle determine the mileage you're likely to get out of your natural gifts. They either squander or preserve your basic genetic endowment.

What does it mean to enjoy a high level of wellness? Beyond the absence of illness and pain, wellness means feeling really alive, with a genuine gusto for life, and having plenty of energy to enjoy it fully. It's a trim, flexible, well-toned body, a twinkle in your eye, and a warm, friendly smile on your face. In short, wellness is the capacity to live your life to its fullest.

On the other hand, over the long term a lack of wellness can lead not only to a loss of trim appearance and vitality, but also to a heightened susceptibility to injury and to many of the major health problems of our time: among them heart and arterial disease, stroke, cancer, diabetes, cirrhosis, emphesema and bronchitis.

The workbook begins with a Lifestyle Inventory which quickly gives you a clear picture of how your current lifestyle patterns are shaping your future well-being. It then provides you with specific information regarding each of these wellness-related lifestyle factors in a concise yet comprehensive statement of the essentials of healthful living. And finally, the workbook introduces you to a completely personalized Positive Lifestyling program which allows you to gradually incorporate these optimal patterns of living into your own way of life, starting from wherever you are right now.

Positive Lifestyling is designed to enhance virtually every facet of your experience, including your physical, emotional, intellectual and intuitive functioning. As you progress in the practice of Positive Lifestyling, you're likely to notice that you're enjoying a greater measure of fulfillment in many important areas: your family life, your social interactions, your professional attainment, as well as your artistic, cultural and other recreational pursuits. That's because your capacity for effective performance in every arena is directly supported by your overall level of well-being.

Discover just how easy it really can be to make well-informed decisions today that maintain your strength, vitality and productivity for the rest of your life. Begin now to tap the fountain of youth that is hidden within you.

LIFESTYLE INVENTORY

HOW YOU SEE YOURSELF

Take a look at the chart below.

From top to bottom, the scale ranges from what you might consider to be your ideal state of health, fitness and well-being, at + 10, to a minimum state of wellness at − 10.

Mark the point on the scale to the right which you feel best represents your overall condition today — that is, your present state of wellness and vitality.

Next, think back in time to a period about five years ago. Get an image of your condition at that time. Now mark the point on the scale to the left which you feel best represents your overall condition as of five years ago.

Connect these two points with an arrow directed from your past to your present condition. This arrow indicates the direction of your recent health history as you have experienced it.

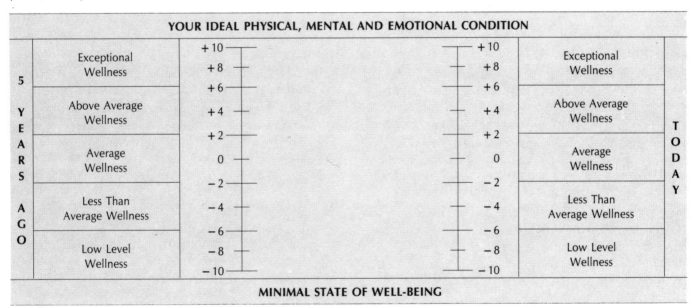

The Lifestyle Inventory will assist you to project a greater measure of wellness into your future.

MEASURE YOUR PRESENT CONDITION

Your Body Composition

The average person, if he or she is in good physical condition at the time, will achieve a desirable weight between the ages of 18 and 23. With this in mind, estimate how many pounds, if any, you are overweight now. If you believe you were overweight during that period, simply give your best estimate.

YOUR PRESENT WEIGHT _____

DIVIDED BY YOUR IDEAL WEIGHT ÷ _____

EQUALS = _____

MINUS − 1.00

EQUALS PERCENT OVERWEIGHT = _____

Enter the score from the table that matches your percent overweight. _____

YOUR SCORE
from the table

Percent Overweight		Your Score	Your Weight Tends To Support
0		50	Exceptional Wellness
1 to 2		47	Exceptional Wellness
3 to 4		44	
5 to 6		41	Above Average Wellness
7 to 9		38	
10 to 13		35	Average Wellness
14 to 19		32	
20 to 26		29	Less Than Average Wellness
27 to 33		26	
34 to 50		23	Low Level Wellness
over 75		20	

Your Resting Heart Rate

How fast your heart beats when you are at rest indicates how hard your heart has to work simply to maintain your basic body functions. This, in turn, is a useful indicator of the fitness of your heart, lungs, blood and blood vessels.

Your resting heart rate may be measured after you have been sitting or lying in a relaxed state for five minutes or so. To determine your heart rate, place the second and third fingers along the thumb side of the opposite wrist, and count the pulsations for one minute.

YOUR RESTING HEART RATE _____

Enter the score from the table that matches your resting heart rate. _____

YOUR SCORE
from the table

Resting Heart Rate		Your Score	Your Rate Tends To Support
under 50		50	Exceptional Wellness
50 to 54		47	Exceptional Wellness
55 to 59		44	
60 to 64		41	Above Average Wellness
65 to 68		38	
69 to 72		35	Average Wellness
73 to 76		32	
77 to 80		29	Less Than Average Wellness
81 to 84		26	
85 to 88		23	Low Level Wellness
over 88		20	

Your Smoking History

Circle the score beside the one statement that best describes your experience with smoking.

  0 I have never smoked, or I quit smoking more than 15 years ago.

− **1** I quit smoking 10 to 15 years ago.

− **2** I quit smoking 5 to 10 years ago.

− **3** I quit smoking less than 5 years ago.

− **20** I presently smoke 1 to 7 cigarettes per day.

− **23** I presently smoke 8 to 14 cigarettes per day or I smoke cigars or a pipe.

− **26** I presently smoke 15 to 25 cigarettes per day.

− **30** I presently smoke more than 25 cigarettes per day.

Circle the score beside *each* statement that is true for you.

− **2** I have lived with a person who smokes during 2 or more of the past 4 years.

− **2** I have worked in a smoky area during 2 or more of the past 4 years.

− **1** I have lived in a high smog area during 2 or more of the past 4 years.

Add up your smoking history scores and enter the total here. − _____

YOUR SCORE

SUMMARIZE YOUR PRESENT CONDITION

Summarize your Present Condition by adding up the three scores you've developed so far.

Your BODY COMPOSITION SCORE   + _____

PLUS: Your RESTING HEART RATE SCORE   + _____

EQUALS: Subtotal   = _____

MINUS: Your SMOKING HISTORY SCORE   − _____

YOUR PRESENT CONDITION SCORE   = _____

Mark Your Score Here	Your Patterns Tend To Support
	Exceptional Wellness
86	Above Average Wellness
72	Average Wellness
58	Less Than Average Wellness
44	Low Level Wellness

The sections to follow explore a number of ways in which your Present Condition is being shaped by your lifestyle.

ENJOY
WELLNESS
FOR LIFE

MEASURE YOUR LIFESTYLE

Your Physical Activity Patterns

For each of the following questions, mark one of the squares that appear beside the single answer that is most correct for you at this time. (Two columns of square are provided so that you can note your responses on two separate occasions. On each such occasion, be sure to mark all of your answers in the same column.)

FULL-BODY STRETCHES

I perform full-body stretches to maintain my flexibility and range of motion:

☐ ☐ **20**   once a week or less.

☐ ☐ **40**   every few days.

☐ ☐ **60**   almost every day.

BODY-TONING

I engage in activities which help me to maintain the tone and strength of my major muscles and bones:

☐ ☐ **10**   once a week or less.

☐ ☐ **20**   one or two times a week.

☐ ☐ **30**   three or more times each week.

CARDIO-RESPIRATORY ACTIVITY

An "aerobic workout" consists of five essential parts:

    first, a brief pre-exercise stretch;
    second, a short warm-up period;
    third, at least 12 minutes of continuous activity which is sufficiently vigorous to maintain your heart rate at 80 percent of its maximum for your age;
    fourth, a short cool-down period; and
    fifth, a brief post-exercise stretch.

I provide my body with a complete, five-part aerobic workout:

☐ ☐ **40**   once a week or less.

☐ ☐ **80**   two or three times a week.

☐ ☐ **120**   more than three times a week.

Add up your physical activity scores for your current set of responses and enter the total here:

YOUR PHYSICAL ACTIVITY SCORE _____ _____

Mark Your Score Here		Your Patterns Tend To Support:
170		Exceptional Wellness
		Above Average Wellness
140		
		Average Wellness
110		
		Less Than Average Wellness
80		
		Low Level Wellness

Your Nutritional Patterns

EATING INDEPENDENCE

I feel that the quantity of food I eat *at meals* is:

☐ ☐ **10** frequent excessive – I usually don't stop eating until I feel full.

☐ ☐ **20** occasionally excessive.

☐ ☐ **30** rarely excessive – I usually finish eating before feeling full.

I feel that the eating and drinking I do – *aside from meals* – is:

☐ ☐ **10** frequent; substantial; high fat or sugar.

☐ ☐ **20** occasional; moderate.

☐ ☐ **30** infrequent; insubstantial; unrefined carbohydrates.

UNREFINED CARBOHYDRATES INTAKE

I eat fresh fruit:

☐ ☐ **5** infrequently – many days none at all.

☐ ☐ **10** occasionally – many days I get some.

☐ ☐ **15** once or twice almost every day.

I eat leafy green vegetables:

☐ ☐ **10** infrequently – many days none at all.

☐ ☐ **20** occasionally – many days I get some.

☐ ☐ **30** once or twice almost every day.

I eat other vegetables such as beans, potatoes, peas, lentils, squash and yams.

☐ ☐ **5** infrequently – many days none at all.

☐ ☐ **10** occasionally – many days I get some.

☐ ☐ **15** almost every day.

The wheat and other grains I eat are mostly:

☐ ☐ **5** highly processed, bleached white.

☐ ☐ **10** medium processed, enriched whole wheat.

☐ ☐ **15** coarse ground, whole grain.

FAT INTAKE

The meats that I eat are mostly:

☐ ☐ **10** high fat – pork, prime beef, hamburger, organ meats, duck, lamb, etc.

☐ ☐ **20** medium fat – lean beef, veal, chicken and turkey with skin.

☐ ☐ **30** lean – fish, chicken and turkey without skin, or no meat at all.

The dairy products that I consume are mostly:

☐ ☐ **5** high fat – whole milk, cream, cheddar and other full-fat cheeses.

☐ ☐ **10** low fat.

☐ ☐ **15** skim milk, low fat cheeses, or no dairy products at all.

I eat deep-fried foods, including most fast foods:

☐ ☐ **5** often – three or more times a week.

☐ ☐ **10** occasionally – about twice a week.

☐ ☐ **15** seldom – once a week or less.

Regarding fats such as butter, margarine, mayonnaise, salad dressings and oils:

☐ ☐ **5** I don't control my intake.

☐ ☐ **10** I eat 3 or 4 teaspoons per day.

☐ ☐ **15** I eat 2 teaspoons or less per day.

Add up your nutritional scores for your current set of responses and enter the total here:

YOUR NUTRITIONAL SCORE _____ _____

Mark Your Score Here		Your Patterns Tend To Support:
		Exceptional Wellness
170		Above Average Wellness
140		Average Wellness
110		Less Than Average Wellness
80		Low Level Wellness

Your Stress Management Patterns

CLARITY AND PERSONAL ORGANIZATION

In my present life situation:

☐ ☐ **3** I feel confined and unable to express myself as I would like.

☐ ☐ **6** I feel somewhat limited.

☐ ☐ **9** I am able to be the person I choose to be, and to do the things I enjoy most.

In areas where I have expectations:

☐ ☐ **3** in one or more key matters, I frequently fear undesired outcomes.

☐ ☐ **6** my expectations are sometimes clouded with doubt regarding my ability to be, do or have as I would like.

☐ ☐ **9** In general, I clearly see myself thinking, feeling and behaving just as I most truly choose to be.

When I feel that I have been slighted, offended or somehow harmed by the actions of another:

☐ ☐ **3** I tend to remain angry, resentful and bitter, hoping that somehow the score can be evened.

☐ ☐ **6** I generally excuse others for their errors and omissions, chalking it up to their ignorance or incompetence.

☐ ☐ **9** I consistently choose to unconditionally forgive any harmful words or actions by others, thus freeing myself for fully effective action, unburdened by blameful thoughts or destructive emotions.

When working on tasks which demand concentration:

☐ ☐ **3** I am frequently distracted by other matters.

☐ ☐ **6** I have some difficulty staying focused on what I'm doing.

☐ ☐ **9** I can usually stay focused on what I'm doing without undue distraction.

Regarding my sense of responsibility:

☐ ☐ **3** I generally feel responsible for everything that is going on.

☐ ☐ **6** I often feel responsible for situations and events that are beyond my control.

☐ ☐ **9** I feel responsible for assuring that my thoughts, feelings and behavior represent me at my very best, and that my conduct is fully harmonized with my values, intuitions and most noble intentions.

ATTITUDE CONTROL

Regarding personal achievement, I am:

☐ ☐ **3** constantly driven to work harder in order to measure up to my own high standards.

☐ ☐ **6** somewhat pressured to work harder in order to prove myself.

☐ ☐ **9** relaxed, confident that I am responding appropriately to my circumstances.

When I am working against a tight schedule:

☐ ☐ **3** I am often nervous, and frequently become impatient with delays.

☐ ☐ **6** I am sometimes nervous, and occasionally become impatient with delays.

☐ ☐ **9** I generally remain calm, responding to delays with patience and renewed determination.

Regarding my need for information:

☐ ☐ **3** I become very uncomfortable when I don't know exactly what is going on.

☐ ☐ **6** I feel somewhat uncomfortable with uncertainty and try hard to eliminate the unknowns.

☐ ☐ **9** I can live with uncertainty, even enjoying the adventure of facing the unknown.

When the assistance of others could aid me in getting my needs met:

- ☐ ☐ 3 I often expect them to be unresponsive to me, and may not even bother to request their help.
- ☐ ☐ 6 I often expect others to be at least somewhat reluctant to assist me, and plan to get what I want through pleading, trickery, intimidation or force.
- ☐ ☐ 9 I generally expect others to be supportive and cooperative once I have brought my needs to their attention.

My satisfaction and sense of accomplishment are derived from:

- ☐ ☐ 3 mainly the rewards and recognition I receive from others.
- ☐ ☐ 6 sometimes my own appreciation; more often the recognition I receive from others.
- ☐ ☐ 9 mainly the personal knowledge that I have performed to be best of my ability.

My interests are:

- ☐ ☐ 3 mostly confined to matters which are related to my work.
- ☐ ☐ 6 somewhat varied.
- ☐ ☐ 9 numerous and varied, including areas that are quite unrelated to my work.

With regard to expressing my feelings:

- ☐ ☐ 3 I keep my true feelings to myself in most situations.
- ☐ ☐ 6 I find it somewhat difficult to express my real feelings.
- ☐ ☐ 9 I find it easy to express my feelings in most situations.

In dealing with my deepest personal concerns.

- ☐ ☐ 3 I feel unable to discuss my most difficult problems with anyone.
- ☐ ☐ 6 sometimes I feel I have no one to talk with about what's really bothering me.
- ☐ ☐ 9 I have trusted persons with whom I can usually discuss whatever is on my mind.

When others are speaking to me:

- ☐ ☐ 3 I'm often thinking of what I'm going to say next, and frequently interrupt the speaker.
- ☐ ☐ 6 I listen intermittently, sometimes interrupting the speaker with my own thoughts.
- ☐ ☐ 9 I usually listen attentively, rarely interrupting the speaker.

The quality of my sleep is:

- ☐ ☐ 3 often disturbed by anxious thoughts or distressing dreams.
- ☐ ☐ 6 sometimes sound; other times disturbed.
- ☐ ☐ 9 sound, peaceful and refreshing; undisturbed by the concerns of the day.

CONSCIOUS RELAXATION

I reduce the effect of stress in my life by engaging in some method of conscious relaxation:

- ☐ ☐ 25 infrequently – once a week or less.
- ☐ ☐ 50 occasionally – every few days.
- ☐ ☐ 75 almost every day.

Add up your stress management scores for your current set of responses and enter the total here.

YOUR STRESS MANAGEMENT SCORE _____ _____

Mark Your Score Here		Your Patterns Tend To Support:
		Exceptional Wellness
168		Above Average Wellness
140		Average Wellness
112		Less Than Average Wellness
84		Low Level Wellness

Chemical Independence

CAFFEINE

My average daily consumption of caffeine drinks, including coffee, non-herbal tea, cocoa, cola and chocolate is:

☐ ☐ **0** one cup or less.

☐ ☐ **− 5** two or three cups.

☐ ☐ **− 10** four or more cups.

ALCOHOL

The amount of alcohol I consume averages:

☐ ☐ **0** one standard serving per day or less of any alcoholic beverage.

☐ ☐ **− 10** two standard servings per day.

☐ ☐ **− 40** three or more standard servings per day.

DRUG INDEPENDENCE

I use other mood altering substances:

☐ ☐ **0** seldom or never.

☐ ☐ **− 10** occasionally − less than once a week.

☐ ☐ **− 20** frequently − once a week or more.

With regard to both prescription and over-the-counter medications:

☐ ☐ **0** I take as little as possible, and then only as directed.

☐ ☐ **− 10** I take quite a bit, sometimes simply for "extra insurance."

☐ ☐ **− 20** I take a lot, whether or not it is clearly necessary at the time; or, I take them in unapproved combinations.

TOBACCO

With regard to tobacco:

☐ ☐ **0** I am a non-smoker.

☐ ☐ **− 50** I use tobacco.

Add up your chemical independence scores for your current set of responses and enter the total here.

YOUR CHEMICAL INDEPENDENCE SCORE _____ _____

Mark Your Score Here			Your Patterns Tend To Support:
0			Exceptional Wellness
0			Above Average Wellness
−18			Average Wellness
−25			Less Than Average Wellness
			Low Level Wellness

Summarize Your Lifestyle

Summarize your Lifestyle Inventory by adding up your total scores from the preceding lifestyle measurements.

Your PHYSICAL ACTIVITY SCORE (from page 6) + _____ + _____

PLUS: Your NUTRITIONAL SCORE (from page 7) + _____ + _____

PLUS: Your STRESS MANAGEMENT SCORE (from page 9) + _____ + _____

EQUALS: Subtotal = _____ = _____

MINUS: Your CHEMICAL INDEPENDENCE SCORE (from page 10) − _____ − _____

YOUR LIFESTYLE SCORE = _____ = _____

Then enter your
PRESENT CONDITION SCORE
(from page 5)

_____

Your Present Condition Score Supports	Your Present Condition Score		Your Lifestyle Score	Your Lifestyle Score Supports
Exceptional Wellness	93		547	Exceptional Wellness
	86		503	
Above Average Wellness	79		464	Above Average Wellness
	72		419	
Average Wellness	65		366	Average Wellness
	58		336	
Less Than Average Wellness	51		274	Less Than Average Wellness
	44		225	
Low Level Wellness	37		67	Low Level Wellness

Place a mark representing your PRESENT CONDITION SCORE on the scale to the left.

Place a second mark, representing your LIFESTYLE SCORE, on the scale to the right.

Connect these two points with an arrow pointing from your PRESENT CONDITION mark to your LIFESTYLE mark.

This arrow gives a general indication of the influence your present lifestyle might be expected to exert on your level of wellness with the passage of time.

Your wellness can be maintained and improved by developing these key factors in your lifestyle:

PROPER PHYSICAL ACTIVITY

BALANCED NUTRITIONAL INTAKE

EFFECTIVE STRESS MANAGEMENT

POSITIVE WEIGHT CONTROL

CHEMICAL INDEPENDENCE

Each of these factors is considered in the sections which follow.

Consult with your physician to develop a more comprehensive picture of your present condition, and to establish a safe and effective strategy for improving your state of health.

Now that you've had a look at your living patterns and how they relate to your wellness, where do you go from here?

The remainder of this workbook is designed to help you answer this question for yourself. It provides information related to each of the lifestyle factors contained in the Inventory, and offers an opportunity for you to design an enjoyable, wellness-oriented personal lifestyle for yourself.

A simple formula for success. Your wellness is largely determined by your lifestyle. Simply by exercising properly for 1 hour every other day, eating and drinking well, and not smoking or misusing drugs, you may raise your physical, mental and emotional efficiency 20-50 percent, increase your energy production 50-200 percent, and greatly reduce your risk of ill-health.

Simply stated, the three basic elements of an effective personal wellness program are:

　1. Regularly engage in concentrated physical activity which utilizes the full range of your physical potential.

　2. Continually balance your nutritional intake against your current activity level and your changing body composition.

　3. Respond to the stressors in your life in potentially fulfilling ways.

Wellness is your heritage.

Your body is the product of perhaps 40,000 generations of human development. If you were born into any but the last two or three of these generations, odds are your lifestyle would be far more active than it is now. For the most part, your food would be fresh, close to its naturally grown state. And your survival would depend as much upon your physical prowess as upon your social skills and mental agility. Throughout this formative period, strength, mobility and endurance were essential to the continuance of life, and fitness was an inevitable by-product of being alive.

Not so today. For people in many areas of the modern world, the recent explosive development of complex social systems, agriculture, science and technology has nearly eliminated the physical exertion of work, as well as the threat of immediate food shortages. This affluence presents the new and demanding challenge of maintaining your personal wellness in a culture which makes few physical demands and which presses on all sides with an abundance of over-rich, over-processed foods. You are now presented with a choice of lifestyles, not all of which assure the maintenance of your personal wellness.

A lack of wellness is often at the root of common problems such as:

　a lack of energy and vitality
　looking and feeling out of shape
　difficulty coping with daily pressures
　nagging aches and pains
　over- or under-weight
　shortness of breath
　frequent minor illnesses
　loss of muscle tone
　persistent lower back pain
　diminished work performance
　difficulty concentrating
　more frequent emotional upsets
　lowered endurance
　limited flexibility
　greater susceptibility to accidents

The effects of your lifestyle are cumulative, increasingly determining the form, composition and functional effectiveness of your body. In general, the younger you are, the less apparent the effects of your lifestyle will be. As you grow older, your body is slowly shaped by the patterns of your experience, and the physical effects of your lifestyle become more pronounced. The living patterns which keep you well also help you to retain your youthful appearance, vitality and general state of fitness.

So what is wellness anyway? Wellness is a quality of life. It's having the personal energy you need to look and feel well, fulfill your responsibilities, effectively handle emergencies, and actively pursue your social, economic, cultural and recreational interests.

No matter who you are or what you do, being well has a positive influence on virtually every aspect of your life — on how you look, how you feel, how you see yourself, and how you perform from day to day.

And over the long haul, a lack of wellness leads to degeneration of critical body functions, greatly increasing the risk of major disease and eventual loss of ability.

It doesn't matter how old you are, what shape you're in now, or how long it's been since you were last active. Nearly everyone can be well with surprisingly little effort.

Your wellness is clearly not a matter of right or wrong, good or bad, should or shouldn't. It **is** a matter of making **intelligent choices**. Choices based upon **the best available information** regarding the effects of your behavior on your personal health and well-being. This workbook, therefore, deliberately avoids the implication that you should or should not do anything. Rather, it recognizes **your ability to shape your own lifestyle**; your ability to make choices that reflect your present level of knowledge. By choosing wellness, you are opening the door to an even more enjoyable and rewarding life.

The chart below lists the major lifestyle factors affecting your wellness, and briefly summarizes the behavioral choices associated with more and less healthful lifestyles.

MORE HEALTHFUL LIFESTYLE	LIFESTYLE FACTORS	LESS HEALTHFUL LIFESTYLE
Regular use of your full physical potential.	Physical Activity	General inactivity.
Low fat, unprocessed carbohydrates and protein balanced with your level of physical activity.	Nutritional Intake	High fat, refined carbohydrates and protein taken in excess of your caloric requirements.
High volume of clean air.	Oxygen Intake	Low volume; smoky, polluted air.
Infrequent use; low quantity.	Alcohol Intake	Frequent use; high quantity.
Minimal use; only as required and as directed.	Drug Intake	Frequent unnecessary use; other than as directed.
Regular, purposeful release of tension.	Stress Management	Chronic unrelieved tension.

PHYSICAL ACTIVITY

III

THE PRINCIPLES OF EXERCISE

Your body — the hundred trillion celled organism supporting your personal awareness — has amazing potential for movement and manipulation of its environment. It's up to you to actualize this potential, for without regular use, your body tends to become stiff, weak, and sluggish. While these are often viewed as the inevitable consequences of aging, proper physical activity can help to reduce the decline of your strength, flexibility and endurance to less than 15 percent between the ages of 20 and 60. And if you were out of shape at 20, you may actually be stronger at 60.

Your body directly reflects the demands which you place upon it. Each day billions of your body cells die and billions more are produced according to the demands of your current activity patterns and the quality of your nutritional intake.

A fully effective exercise program activates three distinct physical potentials: your muscle and joint flexibility, your cardio-respiratory capacity, and the strength and balance of your muscles and bones.

Flexibility

The first component of a well-rounded program of physical activity is full-body stretching. Everyone is familiar with the richly satisfying feeling of a good stretch after a prolonged period of physical inactivity. **You can easily maintain your flexibility and range of motion with a simple routine of regular, systematic stretching.** At least once each day, perhaps upon arising in the morning, take the ten minutes or so needed to give your body a complete stretch. Specific stretching exercises to help you cover all your major joints and muscles are provided on pages 20 and 21.

The key to successful physical development in all areas is progression. In the case of stretching, this means extending and flexing your muscles and joints only to the limits of your personal comfort — never beyond. Perform your stretches in a slow, gentle manner. Breathe deeply while stretching, letting go of a little more tension with each exhalation. You'll be amazed at how your flexibility increases with regular, patient, easy stretching.

Cardio-Respiratory Capacity

The second component of an effective exercise program maintains and expands your cardio-respiratory capacity.

Each of your cells needs a constant supply of fuel and oxygen to give you the energy and stamina you need to get the most out of life. Your body is renewed and energized by the efficient operation of the system that feeds your cells — the cardio-respiratory system composed of your lungs, heart, blood and blood vessels. The more efficiently oxygen is absorbed into your bloodstream and transported throughout your body, the more work you can accomplish with the same expenditure of energy.

Your heart, like any other muscle, tends to lose strength and tone when it is not regularly exercised with sufficient intensity. The rate at which this loss occurs depends upon a number of factors, including the way you eat, how you handle stress, your use of tobacco and alcohol, as well as your basic genetic make-up.

On the other hand, the health and efficiency of your cardio-respiratory system can be maintained and increased by making improvements in these areas, and by a program of regular aerobic activity (aerobic means "with oxygen").

Your lungs are a honeycomb of passages opening to a thousand square feet of surface area — .20 times more than your outer skin. This gives your blood exposure to the atmosphere, so it can exhaust waste carbon dioxide and absorb fresh oxygen.

Your heart pumps more than 5 quarts of blood every minute; 2,000 gallons a day in 10,000 pulsations. The unfit system requires the heart to work 20-30 percent harder just to meet minimal demands. In a year that's 10 million extra beats by an engine that has to last a lifetime.

Your blood vessels are a 60,000 mile labyrinth of tubing distributed throughout your body. When elastic and unobstructed, they can channel blood at speeds up to 50 miles per hour.

Your bloodstream is refreshed with a billion new red blood cells every day. The continued health of your heart and blood vessels depends upon maintaining a balance among certain blood components. For example, too much of the wrong kind of fat clogs the pores in the artery walls, eventually building up layers of plaque which limit the flow of vital fluids.

Aerobic exercise elevates your heart rate to between 70 and 80 percent of its maximum for your age, and keeps it there for at least 12 minutes, and preferably for 30 minutes or more, at a time. Ideally it is acccomplished every day, and it's best not to allow two days to go by without an aerobic workout.

A precautionary note taken from guidelines provided by the National Heart, Lung & Blood Institute: If you are not accustomed to vigorous exercise, and if any of these conditions apply to you, talk with your physician before starting your exercise program:

— heart trouble, heart murmur, or previous heart attack.

— frequent pains or pressure, when exercising, in the left or mid-chest area, left neck, shoulder or arm.

— frequent faintness or dizziness.

— extreme breathlessness after mild exertion.

— uncontrolled high blood pressure or unknown blood pressure.

— bone or joint problems such as arthritis.

— over age 60.

— family history of premature coronary artery disease.

— any other health condition which might need special attention when exercising. (For example, insulin-dependent diabetes.)

THE FIVE PRINCIPLES OF A SAFE AND EFFECTIVE EXERCISE PROGRAM

I. Range	Muscle & Joint Flexibility	Cardio-Respiratory Capacity	Muscle/Bone Balance & Strength
II. Intensity	Execute a full range of possible motions for each of your major joints and muscles.	Engage in continuous activity at your age-adjusted target heart rate.	Selectively exert each of your major muscles.
III. Duration	15 to 30 seconds per movement (9-12 minutes total).	Build from 10 minutes or less to at least ½ hour.	8 to 12 repetitions per muscle (15-20 minutes total).
IV. Frequency	Not less than once a day.	Daily if possible, and not less than every other day.	Every other day, or not less than twice a week.
V. Progression	Extend your range of motion as your flexibility increases.	Gradually intensify your activity while maintaining your target heart rate.	Increase resistance as your strength develops.

A fully effective exercise program activates three distinct physical potentials

Your aerobic exercise may consist of walking, jogging, running, jumping rope, trampolining, bicycling, skating, swimming, rowing, dancercise, cross-country skiing, or possibly courtsports as long as they are sufficiently continuous to maintain your desired exercise heart rate. Activities which involve a lot of starting and stopping usually don't work for this purpose.

Many people enjoy working out with a friend. Sometimes it's difficult to do this while maintaining the proper exercise intensity. Do not attempt to maintain someone else's pace. If necessary, go your own way during your workout, and get together again later.

Pre-exercise stretch.

To minimize your risk of pulling a muscle, begin your aerobic workout with a few simple stretches as shown on pages 20 and 21.

Warm-up.

Following your stretches, and prior to your full-blown exercise, give yourself 5 minutes of cardio-vascular warm-up, performing the same activity you will use for your more vigorous workout. Warm-up is important to open the arterial pathways of your heart, and should be vigorous enough to produce a heart rate approximately 10 to 20 beats per minute slower than your full exercise rate.

Aerobic workout.

Following your warm-up, bring the intensity of your exercise up to a level that sustains your intended heart rate. In the beginning, keep your heart rate at the low end of the target training range — 70% of your age-adjusted maximum heart rate. If this level feels like too much of an exertion for you, begin even lower, perhaps at 60%, and stay at that level for the first two weeks. Then increase it to 65% for a week, then to 70% for a week, and so on until you can comfortably maintain 80% of your maximum. There's no need to rush. Your exercise should never be painful. With easy progression, you'll soon be safely back in good condition.

At first the duration of your workout may be short — perhaps only 3 to 5 minutes. As you build your endurance you'll be able to lengthen your workout to 12, 20, then 30 minutes or more.

Cool-down.

During aerobic exercise, your blood becomes widely distributed throughout your body, and its return to your heart is assisted by the motion of your muscles. If you stop your activity abruptly, your heart may have difficulty handling the circulation on its own, and "blood pooling" may occur, resulting in mild shock, hyperventilation or muscle cramping. A 5 minute cool-down or slowing of your activity to a heart rate which is a few beats slower than your warmup rate will minimize the likelihood of such problems.

Post-exercise stretch.

After aerobic exercise, your rear thigh muscles and lower back muscles may shorten, producing an abnormal pelvic tilt which is often accompanied by low back pain. Performing the post-exercise stretches specified on page 21 will help you to avoid this problem.

Some potential benefits of a well-designed exercise program are: greater strength, endurance, flexibility and vitality; reduced muscle tension, anxiety, depression, boredom and mental fatigue; improved muscle tone, bone density; metabolism and weight control; reduced risk of heart and arterial disease, low back pain and sleep disorders; increased productivity and greater enjoyment of work; as well as an enhanced sense of well-being and self-confidence. Indeed, proper physical activity can add a lot to the quality of your life, and inactivity can take a heavy toll.

Your target heart rate.

To assure that you are maintaining the correct exercise intensity, you must be able to monitor your heart rate during exercise. Heart rate is best determined by placing the second and third fingers along the thumb side of the opposite wrist, and counting the pulsations for ten seconds.

While exercising, stop periodically and take a ten-second count. It is important to quickly determine your exercise heart rate before the slower recovery rate commences. If you find that your heart rate is below the rate you have selected for your workout, increase the speed or intensity of your activity. Then, after a minute or so, take another count and adjust your intensity accordingly. If your heart rate is above your intended rate, continue your exercise, reducing the intensity a bit until you can maintain the desired rate.

A note about exceeding the target rate: it may seem that if 80% of your maximum is good, then 90% might be even better. This is not the case. Above 80% of the maximum rate for your age, your activity may become "anaerobic" — that is, your body may not be able to support the activity over an extended period, resulting in early exhaustion. Aerobic activity is accomplished at a level which you could maintain for hours if necessary, without becoming totally exhausted. Sprinting and weight lifting are anaerobic activities in that they intentionally press the body to the limits of its capability over a short span of time. While this may build muscle mass, it does not provide an adequate cardio-vascular workout.

One of the first steps to take in getting started in your exercise program is obtaining the proper equipment. A good pair of running shoes, for example, is essential to protecting yourself from possible injury.

The table below provides age-adjusted maximum heart rates and target training rates as well as a conversion to the ten second count.

EXERCISE TRAINING RANGE

Age	Maximum Attainable Heart Rate (beats/min)	Training Range (70-80% of max)	Target 10 Second Training Range
20	200	140-160	23-27
25	195	136-156	22-26
30	190	133-152	22-25
35	185	129-148	21-25
40	180	126-144	21-24
45	175	122-140	20-23
50	170	119-136	20-23
55	165	115-132	19-22
60	160	112-128	19-21
65	155	108-124	18-21

Muscle/Bone Balance, Tone and Strength

The third component of an effective physical activity program is body toning, which **develops the strength, symmetry and balance of your muscle and bone structure.** This kind of exercise is not intended to build "bulging" muscles, although you can use it to add muscle mass if that is desired. Rather, it is designed to **prevent the reduction of bone density and muscle mass which tends to occur when your strength is not used.**

Without sufficient use, significant loss of bone may begin at about age 30 for women, and age 50 for men. With passing years of inactivity, the bones may gradually weaken, raising the risk of easy breakage. An adequate intake of calcium is also essential to maintaining bone density.

You can maintain your body tone in just 2 or 3 short sessions per week of 15 to 20 minutes each. The methods which may be used include a variety of excellent mechanical systems, free weights, isometrics and slimnastics. Body toning exercises are given on pages 22 and 23. Stretch out tightened muscles after your toning exercises.

It's important to remember that body toning is not likely to give you a complete aerobic workout, and it is not a substitute for stretching. Each of these is a distinct, yet complementary, activity. If you're short of time one day, choose first your stretches and aerobic workout. The benefits are more fundamental and immediate, and these capacities diminish more rapidly when they are not utilized.

WARNING SIGNS

It's important for you to be aware of the common warning signs related to heart trouble. If you experience any of these symptoms, see your physician: chest pains, pain down arms, especially the left arm, swelling of ankles or hands, purple fingertips, or light headedness.

CALORIE EXPENDITURE CHART

Activity raises the body heat, or metabolic rate. This elevated body heat burns off calories not only during the period of activity itself, but also for several hours afterwards. This chart gives a rough approximation of the calories expended in selected activities by a person weighing 150 pounds. Proportionally more will be expended for additional body weight, and less for lower body weight.

Activity	Calories Per Minute
Dancing —	
Ballroom	5.4
Dancercise	7.0
Disco	6.5
Slow	4.4
Square or round	6.0
Gardening —	
General	3.8
Lawn mowing (hand mower)	7.7
Planting seedlings	4.8
Raking	5.4
General Activities —	
Driving a car	2.8
Eating	1.7
Lying at ease	1.5
Sex	7.2
Sitting quietly	1.7
Sleeping (basal metabolism)	1.0
Standing quietly	1.7
Walking — 17 min./mile	5.4
Housekeeping Tasks —	
Bed-making	3.9
Carpet cleaning	3.5
Cooking	3.5
Food Shopping	4.5
Ironing	2.7
Knitting/Sewing	1.8
Mopping floor	4.8
Scrubbing floors (vigorously)	12.0
Occupational Activity —	
Bricklaying	4.0
Carpentry	6.8
Desk work — general	2.2
typing	1.8
Farm work in field	7.3
Painting at an easel	2.0
Piano playing	3.2
Sports/Athletics —	
Archery	2.8
Badminton — singles	5.6
Basketball — full court	12.0
half court	5.0
Bowling	3.5

Activity	Calories Per Minute
Sports/Athletics (continued) —	
Calisthenics	5.2
Canoeing — 15 min./mile	6.9
Circuit training	5.5
Cycling — 5 min./mile	10.6
casual	4.6
Golf — foursome carrying clubs	6.0
walking without clubs	4.6
with cart	3.4
Gymnastics	5.2
Handball	10.9
Hiking — without load	5.0
with 40 lb. backpack	6.8
climbing without load	9.5
climbing with 10 lb. load	10.1
Horseback riding — trot	8.0
walk	4.0
Interval training	10.8
Judo/karate	5.2
Mountain climbing	9.5
Racquetball	10.0
Roller skating — speed	11.2
casual	5.8
Rope-skipping — 80 turns/min.	13.3
Running — 6 min./mile	16.2
jogging 8 min./mile	12.6
Skating — high speed	15.0
casual	5.8
Skiing — cross country	11.6
down-hill (vigorously)	9.5
Skin diving	10.0
Soccer	12.0
Softball or baseball	4.7
Squash	10.7
Surfing	9.2
Swimming — 50 yds./min.	10.5
casual	5.3
Tennis — singles	6.0
doubles	4.6
table tennis	4.0
Trampolining	5.6
Volleyball — 2 players	9.2
6 players	5.8
Water skiing	7.8
Weight training	7.8

CARDIO-RESPIRATORY EXERCISE PROGRAMS

A WALKING PROGRAM

	Warm Up	Target Zone Exercise	Cool Down	Total Time
Week 1	Walk slowly 5 min.	Walk briskly 5 min.	Walk slowly 5 min.	15 min.
Week 2	Walk slowly 5 min.	Walk briskly 7 min.	Walk slowly 5 min.	17 min.
Week 3	Walk slowly 5 min.	Walk briskly 9 min.	Walk slowly 5 min.	19 min.
Week 4	Walk slowly 5 min.	Walk briskly 11 min.	Walk slowly 5 min.	21 min.
Week 5	Walk slowly 5 min.	Walk briskly 13 min.	Walk slowly 5 min.	23 min.
Week 6	Walk slowly 5 min.	Walk briskly 15 min.	Walk slowly 5 min.	25 min.
Week 7	Walk slowly 5 min.	Walk briskly 18 min.	Walk slowly 5 min.	28 min.
Week 8	Walk slowly 5 min.	Walk briskly 20 min.	Walk slowly 5 min.	30 min.
Week 9	Walk slowly 5 min.	Walk briskly 23 min.	Walk slowly 5 min.	33 min.
Week 10	Walk slowly 5 min.	Walk briskly 26 min.	Walk slowly 5 min.	36 min.
Week 11	Walk slowly 5 min.	Walk briskly 28 min.	Walk slowly 5 min.	38 min.
Week 12	Walk slowly 5 min.	Walk briskly 30 min.	Walk slowly 5 min.	40 min.

Week 13 on:

Check your pulse periodically to be sure you are exercising within your target zone. As you get more in shape, try exercising within the upper range of your heart zone. Remember to enjoy yourself.

If you are over 40 and have not been active, begin with the walking program. After completing the walking program, you can start with week 3 of the jogging program.

A JOGGING PROGRAM

	WARM UP	TARGET ZONE EXERCISING	COOL DOWN	TOTAL TIME
Week 1	Stretch 5 min.	Walk 10 min.	Walk slowly 3 min., stretch 2 min.	20 min.
Week 2	Stretch 5 min., walk 5 min.	Jog 1 min., walk 5 min., jog 1 min.	Walk slowly 3 min., stretch 2 min.	22 min.
Week 3	Stretch 5 min., walk 5 min.	Jog 3 min., walk 5 min., jog 3 min.	Walk slowly 3 min., stretch 2 min.	26 min.
Week 4	Stretch 5 min., walk 4 min.	Jog 5 min., walk 4 min., jog 5 min.	Walk slowly 3 min., stretch 2 min.	28 min.
Week 5	Stretch 5 min., walk 4 min.	Jog 5 min., walk 4 min., jog 5 min.	Walk slowly 3 min., stretch 2 min.	28 min.
Week 6	Stretch 5 min., walk 4 min.	Jog 6 min., walk 4 min., jog 6 min.	Walk slowly 3 min., stretch 2 min.	30 min.
Week 7	Stretch 5 min., walk 4 min.	Jog 7 min., walk 4 min., jog 7 min.	Walk slowly 3 min., stretch 2 min.	32 min.
Week 8	Stretch 5 min., walk 4 min.	Jog 8 min., walk 4 min., jog 8 min.	Walk slowly 3 min., stretch 2 min.	34 min.
Week 9	Stretch 5 min., walk 4 min.	Jog 9 min., walk 4 min., jog 9 min.	Walk slowly 3 min., stretch 2 min.	36 min.
Week 10	Stretch 5 min., walk 4 min.	Jog 13 min.	Walk slowly 3 min., stretch 2 min.	27 min.
Week 11	Stretch 5 min., walk 4 min.	Jog 15 min.	Walk slowly 3 min., stretch 2 min.	29 min.
Week 12	Stretch 5 min., walk 4 min.	Jog 17 min.	Walk slowly 3 min., stretch 2 min.	31 min.
Week 13	Stretch 5 min., walk 2 min., jog slowly 2 min.	Jog 17 min.	Walk slowly 3 min., stretch 2 min.	31 min.
Week 14	Stretch 5 min., walk 1 min., jog slowly 3 min.	Jog 17 min.	Walk slowly 3 min., stretch 2 min.	31 min.
Week 15	Stretch 5 min., jog slowly 3 min.	Jog 17 min.	Walk slowly 3 min., stretch 2 min.	30 min.

Week 16 on:

Check your pulse periodically to see if you are exercising within your target zone. As you become more fit, try exercising within the upper range of your target zone. Remember that your goal is to continue to get the benefits you are seeking, while enjoying your activity. Listen to your body and build up less quickly, if needed.

FULL
BODY
STRETCHES

Execute a full range of possible motions for each of your major joints and muscles, extending the range as your flexibility increases. Perform each exercise for 15 to 30 seconds (9-12 minutes total) once a day. Accomplish the exercises slowly and gently, never bouncing or forcing the movement. Continue to breathe fully and at a normal rate, relaxing a little further into your stretch with each exhalation.

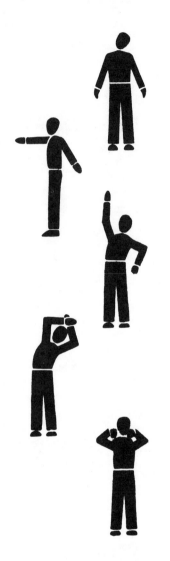

NECK ROTATIONS

Either standing or sitting, rotate your head 5 times in a clockwise direction; then 5 times in a counterclockwise direction.

ARM CIRCLES

While standing, slowly rotate and stretch your arms for 10 seconds as in the backstroke; then reverse the direction of rotation for another 10 seconds.

REACH-UP STRETCH

While standing, stretch and reach toward the ceiling; first with your right arm, then with your left, alternating for 10 times.

SIDE STRETCHER

While standing with your hands clasped above your head, bend to the left and hold for 5 seconds; then bend to the right and hold for 5 seconds. Repeat 6 times.

WAIST TWIST

While standing with your legs bent slightly and your hands on your shoulders, twist your upper body from side to side while keeping your lower body stationary. Continue for 10 full twists.

LEG STRETCHERS

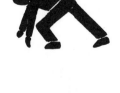

Assuming a sprinter's position, stretch your achilles tendons and calf muscles by pointing your back heel while lowering your hips. Repeat with other leg.

Once again assuming the sprinter's position, stretch your inner thigh muscles by lowering your hips toward floor while allowing your back heel to rise somewhat.

FORWARD BEND

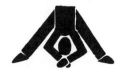

Standing with legs apart, bend forward at the waist, keeping your legs straight. Hold for 10 seconds. Bend knees slightly before returning to standing position.

ANKLE STRETCHES

While sitting with your legs straight and your heels touching the floor, rotate your ankles for 15 seconds in each direction. Then, pointing your toes, fully extend your ankles for 5 seconds. Next, fully flex your ankles for 5 seconds. Repeat 5 times.

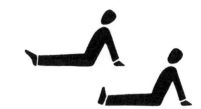

TRUNK FLEXION*

While sitting with your legs extended, and your feet flexed, bend forward for 5 seconds, reaching for your toes. Repeat 5 times.

STRAIGHT LEG PULL*

While sitting with your knees bent, your heels on the floor and your hands grasping your toes, slowly straighten one leg until fully extended, pulling back on the toes — hold for 5 seconds. Then, while returning the straightened leg to a bent position, simultaneously straighten the other leg and hold for 5 seconds. Repeat 5 times.

HURDLERS STRETCH

While sitting with one leg extended and the other turned back, reach forward with both hands for 10 seconds, attempting to touch the extended foot. Repeat with other leg.

SIDE LEG LIFTS

While lying on your side with your legs straight, lift the top leg as high as you can and hold for 2 seconds before lowering. Repeat 20 times, then turn to other side.

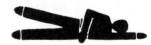

BUTTOCK STRETCH*

While lying on your side, pull your top knee toward your chest. Then relax, slide your hand to your ankle, and pull your ankle toward the rear, stretching the front of your upper leg. Repeat 5 times then turn to other side.

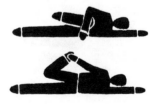

MAD CAT

While on hands and knees, exhale as you arch your spine as high as possible, pulling your chin toward your chest — hold for 5 seconds. Then, as you inhale, bring your head up while lowering your back until it is fully arched in the opposite, sway-back position — hold for 5 seconds. Repeat 6 times.

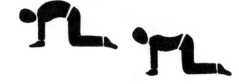

---

* **After aerobic or body toning exercise, stretch out your rear thigh and lower back muscles with these post-exercise stretches. Then finish off with a set of Sit-Ups as shown on page 23.**

BODY TONING

These exercises develop the tone, strength, symmetry and balance of your muscle and bone structure. The methods which may be used to maintain your body tone include isometrics, slimnastics, a variety of mechanical systems such as Nautilus or Total Gym, and free weights. Body toning should be conducted smoothly and rhythmically, inhaling at time of least exertion and exhaling at time of greatest exertion.

To prepare your body for these exercises, perform the stretches given on pages 20 and 21. Then, after you have finished your body toning exercises, stretch out any tightened muscles with the post-exercise stretches indicated on the same pages.

PUSH-UPS

Begin by lying on your stomach with your hands shoulder width apart. Keeping your body rigid, push up until your arms are straight. Then by bending at the elbows, lower your body until you can touch your chin to the floor. Repeat 5-30 times. If this is too difficult, begin by keeping your knees on the floor.

STOMACH FLUTTER KICKS

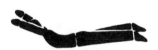

Lying on your stomach with your arms extended above your head, raise your legs and upper torso so that only your stomach is on the floor. Then kick your legs at a comfortable pace for 5-20 seconds.

HIP RAISING

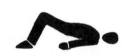

Lying on your back with your hands at your sides and your knees bent, push up, tighten and hold your hips and buttocks for 5-10 seconds, then lower. Repeat 5-15 times.

BACK FLUTTER KICKS

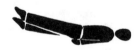

Lying on your back with your hands under your buttocks for support, raise your legs 6 inches from the floor and kick them alternately for 5-20 seconds.

HALF SQUATS

Standing with your hands on your hips, lower your body to a half squat position while thrusting your arms forward, then return to the starting position. Repeat 5-20 times.

Standing with your feet turned outward, lower your body to a half squat while raising your arms sideways, then return to the starting position. Repeat 5 to 20 times.

TOWEL STRETCH

Grasping towel ends, simultaneously extend and flex your arms and shoulders. Use a variety of positions, including above, behind and in front of your head.

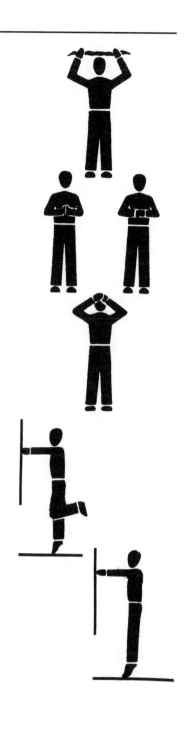

PUSH AND PULL

With your hands opposing each other at chest level, press palms together for 5-10 seconds. Repeat several times. Then grasp your hands or wrists at chest level and pull for 5-10 seconds. Repeat several times.

NECK ISOMETRICS

With your hands on your forehead, keep your neck straight while pushing with slowly increasing pressure until firm neck tension is reached. Hold for 5 seconds. Now put your left hand on the left side of your head and repeat as above. Then put your right hand on the right side of your head and repeat as above. Place both hands on the back of your head and apply pressure backward.

CALF RAISES

Using a wall or chair for balance, stand with feet together and lift right leg slightly. Raise and lower left heel 20 to 50 times. Then lift left leg while raising and lowering right heel 20 to 50 times.

FULL LEG & BUTTOCK TIGHTENING

Standing with hands on wall for balance, raise both heels while tightening calves, thighs and buttocks — hold for 10 to 15 seconds. Then relax for 10 seconds and repeat.

SIT-UPS

While lying flat on your back with knees bent at 45 degrees, arms crossed on chest and stomach muscles pulled in tightly, curl up and forward until shoulders are lifted 5 to 6 inches off the floor; then lower. Without relaxing stomach muscles, curl up and forward again, this time while pointing left shoulder toward right knee; then lower. Continuing to maintain stomach muscle tension, curl up and forward once again while pointing right shoulder toward left knee; then lower. Perform five repetitious of this three step routine to begin with, slowly working up to 20 repetitions (60 total sit-ups). Note that this exercise does not call for curling up to a full sitting position, as this is risky to the lower back, and does not improve strengthening of the stomach muscles.

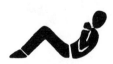

EXERCISES FOR THE LOWER BACK

Seven out of ten adults over the age of 35 suffer from some degree of low back pain, much of it due to two controllable factors: insufficient trunk flexibility and weak abdominal muscles. An imbalance of strength or length between the abdominal muscles and the rear thigh and back muscles may cause an improper pelvic tilt, thus producing a misalignment of the spine with low grade irritation and pain. This condition sometimes occurs when the legs are rapidly strengthened without complementary stretching exercises.

These exercises shorten and strengthen the abdominal muscles while stretching and lengthening the rear thigh and low back muscles.

If you are not experiencing back pain you may begin the intermediate exercises after about a week of preconditioning with the beginning exercises, later adding the advanced.

If you have been suffering with pain in the lower back, then you may experience minor, short-term discomfort while performing some of the exercises. If it does not persist, and does not bother you during subsequent hours, you may want to continue those exercises. **Discontinue immediately any exercise which produces significant or continuing pain.**

The exercises are presented in three parts: beginning, intermediate and advanced. The beginning exercises are more passive, promoting moderate stretching and conditioning. For the first three weeks, these exercises may be performed every other day. If no additional pain is experienced, increase the number of exercise sessions to 4 or 5 days per week for the next three weeks, and to 6 or 7 days per week for the following three weeks. After the ninth week, many people perform the exercises twice each day.

If you have no additional pain following the end of the twelfth week, continue the beginning exercises while carefully adding the intermediate. After several weeks of performing the intermediate exercises, you may add the advanced.

Execute each exercise slowly and gently for at least one minute.

Lower back pain — a troublesome by-product of sedentary living — is experienced by seven out of ten adults over the age of 35. As much as 80 percent of all back pain is related to two controllable factors: trunk flexibility and abdominal strength.

Beginning Exercises

BACK PRESS

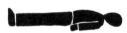

1. Lying flat on back, legs straight.
2. Tighten buttocks muscles, pull stomach muscles in tightly, press lower spine to floor. Hold 10 seconds.
3. Relax for 10 seconds and repeat.

BACK PRESS (knees bent)

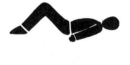

1. Lying flat on back, knees bent at 45 degrees.
2. Tighten buttocks, pull stomach muscles in tightly, pressing lower spine to floor. Hold for 10 seconds.
3. Relax for 10 seconds and repeat.

BACK PRESS (standing)

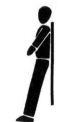

1. Standing, back against wall, heels 5-6 inches from wall, feet 5-6 inches apart, legs straight.
2. Tighten buttocks muscles, pull stomach muscles in tightly, press hips, spine and shoulders against wall. Hold for 15 seconds.
3. Relax for 15 seconds and repeat.

KNEE TO CHEST (buttock stretch)

1. Lying flat on back, legs straight.
2. Pull stomach muscles in tightly, slowly bring one knee towards chest. Grasping front of leg with both hands, pull knee to chest and hold for 5 seconds.
3. Release and straighten leg.
4. Repeat with other leg.

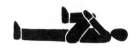

FORWARD SPINE CURL

1. Lying flat on back, knees bent at 45 degrees, arms crossed on chest.
2. Pull stomach muscles in tightly, keep lower spine and pelvis in contact with floor. Slowly curl neck forward until chin comfortably touches chest; continue curling forward until shoulders are lifted up 5-6 inches off of floor. Hold for 5 seconds.
3. Return to starting position and repeat.

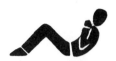

MAD CAT

1. Crawling position, back straight, hands, knees and toes on floor, stomach muscles pulled in tightly.
2. Exhale as you arch your spine as high as comfortably possible, pulling your chin toward chest. Hold for 5 seconds.
3. Then, as you inhale, bring your head up while lowering your back until it is fully arched in the opposite sway-back position. Hold for 5 seconds.
4. Repeat.

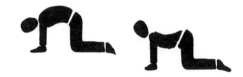

FORWARD LEAN

1. Sitting, knees bent to sides, bottoms of feet touching each other, hands grasping feet.
2. Pulling stomach muscles in tightly, slowly bend forward, comfortably bringing face toward feet. Hold 10 seconds.
3. Return to starting position and repeat.

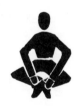

FORWARD TRUNK LEAN

1. Sitting, legs straight, hands grasping back of knees.
2. Pulling stomach muscles in tightly, slowly lean forward, comfortably bringing face toward knees. Hold 10-30 secs.
3. Return to starting position and repeat.

Intermediate Exercises

BACK PRESS (replaces beginning version)

1. While standing straight against a wall, touch as many points as possible — heels, legs, buttocks, spine and head.
2. Pulling stomach and buttocks muscles in tightly, press low spine firmly against wall. Hold for 15 seconds.
3. Relax for 15 seconds and repeat.

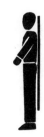

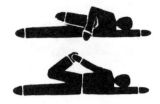

KNEE TO CHEST

1. Lying on side, legs straight.

2. Slowly bring top knee toward chest. Grasping knee with hand, pull inward toward chest. Hold for 10 seconds.

3. Relax tension, sliding hand to ankle. Pull ankle back toward buttock. Hold for 10 seconds. Repeat.

4. Turn over and repeat with other leg.

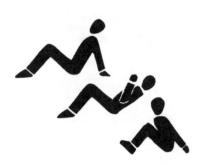

SIT-BACK

1. Sitting, knees bent at 45 degrees.

2. With stomach muscles pulled in tightly and hands folded on chest, slowly sit back until shoulders touch floor (take 4 to 6 seconds to complete this movement).

3. Using elbows and hands to assist, return to starting position. Repeat.

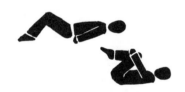

BOTH KNEES TO CHEST

1. Lying on back, knees bent at 45 degrees, arms at sides, hands flat on floor, stomach muscles pulled in tightly.

2. Slowly bring both knees toward chest. Grasping knees with hands, pull toward chest. Hold for 5 seconds.

3. Return to starting position.

4. Rest for 5 seconds and repeat.

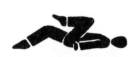

ALTERNATING KNEES TO CHEST

1. Lying on back, knees bent at 45 degrees, spine pressed to floor, stomach muscles pulled in tightly.

2. Bring one knee to chest. Return first knee to starting position while simultaneously bringing other knee to chest. Continue alternating knees to chest for 30 seconds, only briefly touching heel of down foot to floor.

3. Rest for 30 seconds and repeat.

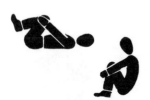

BACK ROLL

1. Lying on back on padded floor, knees bent to chest, ankles crossed, hands holding ankles, stomach muscles pulled in tightly.

2. Curl head forward, simultaneously pulling down on ankles. Gently rock forward and backwards several times, ending in a sitting position.

3. Rest for 5 seconds and repeat.

Advanced Exercises

STRAIGHT LEG PULL

1. Sitting, knees bent, heels on floor, hands grasping toes.
2. Slowly straighten one leg until fully extended, pulling back on toes. Hold for 15 seconds.
3. Return first leg to bent position, simultaneously extending opposite leg. Hold for 15 seconds. Repeat.

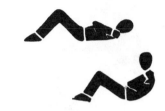

BENT KNEE SHOULDER PULL-UP

1. Lying on back, knees bent, feet wide apart on floor, hands grasping shoulders next to neck.
2. Tightening stomach muscles, curl head and shoulders up, pointing left elbow toward right thigh. Hold 15 secs.
3. Return to starting position and rest for 10 seconds.
4. Repeat, pointing right elbow toward left thigh.
5. Repeat with each elbow.

ISOMETRIC SIT-UP

1. Balancing on buttocks, legs and spine straight, feet and shoulders raised, stomach muscles pulled in tightly.
2. Bend forward at waist, simultaneously bending knees and bringing them toward face. Hold for 5 seconds.
3. Return to starting position and repeat.

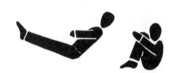

OPPOSITE KNEE SIT-UP

1. Lying on back, knees bent at 45 degrees, hands touching side of head, stomach muscles pulled in tightly.
2. Bending up at waist, simultaneously bring left knee up to touch right elbow.
3. Return to starting position.
4. Repeat, touching right knee to left elbow.
5. Repeat with each knee.

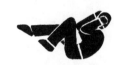

SIDE TILTS

1. Lying on back, knees together and 45 degrees, feet 3 to 5 inches off floor, arms out to side on floor, stomach muscles pulled in tightly.
2. Keeping shoulders, arms, and buttocks flat on floor, tilt knees to right side. Hold for 5 seconds.
3. Return to starting position.
4. Tilt knees to left side. Repeat.

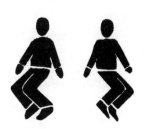

PREVENTIVE EXERCISES FOR LEGS, ANKLES & FEET

Running is common to many aerobic activities, including courtsports, dancercise and jogging. These exercises help to reduce the risk of leg injury.

Exercises for Shin Splints

The term "shin splints" describes pain occurring along the front or sides of the shin bone. Running on very hard surfaces sometimes vibrates the muscles away from the shin bones, producing pain. The following exercises, performed 3 times a day, help to alleviate and prevent shin splints.

WALK FOR DORSIFLEXION (use only if your balance is good)

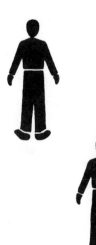

1. Standing, weight on heels, toes lifted from floor.
2. Step with short stride for 50 paces.
3. Rest and repeat 5 times.
4. Perform same exercise with toes turned inward.
5. Perform with toes turned outward.

WALK FOR LATERAL STRETCH

1. Standing, barefoot, weight on sides of feet, toes curled and turned inward.
2. Stepping with short stride, walk 50 paces.
3. Rest and repeat 5 times.

Exercises for Achilles Tendonitis

Pain radiating up the rear heel cord should receive professional attention. Running on your toes, walking upstairs, toe lifts, skipping rope or running in shoes that have insufficient heel counter may produce achilles tendonitis. These stretches are designed to help prevent this injury.

STRAIGHT ANKLE PULL

1. Sitting, knees bent, heels on floor, hands grasping toes.
2. Slowly straighten one leg until fully extended, pulling back on toes. Hold for 5 seconds.
3. Return leg to bent position, simultaneously straightening other leg. Hold for 5 seconds.
4. Repeat for 1 to 3 minutes.

LATERAL ANKLE PULL

1. Sitting, knees bent, heels on floor, hands grasping outside of foot near toes.
2. Slowly straighten one leg until fully extended, pulling back on side of foot. Hold for 5 seconds.
3. Return leg to bent position while extending other leg.
4. Repeat for 1 to 3 minutes.

MEDIAL ANKLE PULL

1. Sitting, knees bent, heels on floor, hands grasping inside border of foot near toes.
2. Slowly straighten one leg until fully extended, pulling back on side of foot. Hold for 5 seconds.
3. Return leg to bent position while extending other leg.
4. Repeat for 1 to 3 minutes.

ACHILLES TENDON STRETCH

1. Standing 3 to 4 feet from wall, hands on wall.
2. Extend one leg back 3 to 4 more feet with heel on floor. Retaining heel-floor contact, bend front knee and move trunk forward slowly toward wall so that rear leg muscles are stretched. Hold for 5 seconds.
3. Repeat with other leg. Continue for 1 to 3 minutes.

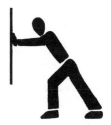

Exercises for Flat Feet

If you have flat feet, in addition to performing these exercises, you may need orthotics or special arch supports.

MARBLE PICK-UP

1. Sitting in chair, barefoot, marble-size paper wads on floor.
2. Pick up pieces of paper by forcefully gripping with toes. Hold for 5 seconds before dropping paper to floor.
3. Repeat with other foot.

TOWEL PULL

1. Sitting in chair, barefoot, towel on floor with 2 to 5 pounds of weight on towel.
2. Gripping towel with toes, pull completely past heel of other foot.
3. Repeat with other foot.

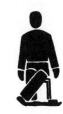

TOWEL SLIDING TO SIDE

1. Sitting in chair, barefoot, towel on floor to side of foot with 2 to 5 pounds of weight on towel.
2. Gripping towel with toes, move completely past toes of other foot.
3. Repeat with other foot.

TOWEL PUSH AWAY

1. Sitting in chair, barefoot, towel on floor behind heels with 2 to 5 pounds of weight on towel.
2. Gripping towel with toes, move completely past toes of other foot.
3. Repeat with other foot.

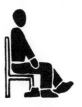

FOODS AND THEIR NUTRITIONAL VALUE

In addition to depending upon a well designed program of physical activity, your continuing wellness is maintained by proper nutrition. Your body needs certain essential nutrients — carbohydrates, protein, fats, vitamins, minerals, water and air. And it needs them in proper quantity, purity and balance to maintain optimal health and well-being.

The primary vehicles for delivering energy and nutrients to your body are: **protein**, mainly from meats, fish and certain vegetables; **carbohydrates**, primarily from plant food sources; and **fats**. To gain their full benefits, your body needs to receive them in amounts that are closely matched to your requirements: no more and no less.

No single food item can provide you with all the nutrients you need for optimal health. In fact, one of the best ways to assure that you're giving your body everything it needs is to eat a variety of good foods. The greater the variety, the less your chance of either a deficiency or an excess of any single nutrient.

The energy in food is considerable, though less noticeable than in some other sources because it is released slowly and at many points in the body. For example, the 375 calorie energy yield of a double dip ice cream cone is equivalent to the explosive power of 1½ sticks of dynamite.

The Basic Food Groups

The easiest and surest way to obtain a balanced variety of good foods is to regularly select from among all the basic food groups. These include:

Carbohydrates

Breads and cereals, including whole grain cereals, rolls, tortillas, noodles, spaghetti, macaroni, pancakes, waffles, muffins, oatmeal, rice, barley, bulgar or cracked wheat.

Leafy green vegetables, including romaine, red and green leaf lettuce, chard, collards and other greens, broccoli, brussel sprouts, cabbage, asparagus, parsley, watercress and scallions.

Fresh fruit and vegetables rich in vitamin C, including citrus fruits, tomatoes, berries, melons, peppers, cabbage, cauliflower, broccoli and brussel sprouts.

Protein

Animal sources, including meats, poultry, seafood and eggs.

Vegetable sources, including dried beans, lentils, split peas, peanuts, peanut butter and other nuts.

Fats

Fats and oils, including butter, margarine, vegetable oils, mayonnaise, salad dressings, cream, seeds, avocadoes, olives and bacon.

Carbohydrates: Quick Energy From Plants

Carbohydrates, chemically the least complex of the major food types, are readily digested into a simple blood sugar called glucose. Glucose fuels your brain activity and other body processes. Your muscles chemically burn glucose, in combination with fat, to release energy for body heat and motion. Carbohydrates carry many of the vitamins and minerals essential to normal body functioning.

Fiber

Most unrefined carbohydrates contain large amounts of plant fiber which, though undigestible in itself, possesses many positive nutritional qualities. It helps you to digest all your foods and speeds the elimination of wastes, reducing the concentrations of cancer promoting substances in your intestines. Many fiber-rich foods decrease fat absorption and reduce blood cholesterol levels. Certain plant fibers also help to detoxify various drugs and chemicals. In addition, fiber has the marvelous quality of making you feel full without adding any calories. And finally, fiber helps you to fend off such problems as heart disease, certain types of cancer, diabetes, hemorrhoids and constipation.

Each person's need for fiber is different. You can tell if you're eating enough fiber-rich food from your stool: if it's soft and floats, you're probably getting enough fiber; if it's hard and sinks, you could probably use more fibrous foods.

Processed Carbohydrates: Sugar

By removing nutrients and fiber from plant food sources to make products like white flour and sugar, large numbers of calories are concentrated into a low bulk form with little nutritional value, and notable digestive disadvantages. They can be eaten quickly, without producing the sense of fullness normally associated with consuming unprocessed foods having a like number of calories. And they are quickly absorbed into your bloodstream, temporarily flooding your system with more fuel than it needs for efficient operation.

Amazingly, 130 pounds of sugar are consumed per person each year in this country. That's about 36 teaspoons of sugar every day! Much of it comes from packaged foods and soft drinks — a 12-ounce can of soda pop contains about 9 teaspoons of sugar. High sugar intake promotes obesity, diabetes, tooth decay and perhaps even heart disease. You may also experience fatigue after consuming a large amount of sugar in something called reactive hypoglycemia. There's little doubt that your body works more efficiently when it's not overloaded with sugar. Sugar is more properly used as a seasoning, in small amounts, than it is as a main ingredient in your food.

Protein: The Body's Building Blocks

Protein is the primary source of building materials for your heart, brain, and other internal organs, as well as for your blood, muscles, skin, hair and nails. Protein also plays an important role in the formation of many essential body chemicals. Your body needs protein, not only for initial growth, but also to replace the billions of cells which die each day and are eliminated.

Over the past century, average protein intake has remained about the same. However, the source of protein has changed. Early in the century, half of the protein came from grains, legumes (peas, beans and lentils), potatoes and other vegetables. The other half came from animal products. Today, a much higher percentage of all the protein consumed comes from animal products. This change toward more animal protein has contributed both to an increase in fat intake and to a decrease in carbohydrate and fiber intake. For example, hamburger is a combination of protein and fat, while pinto beans are a combination of protein, starch and fiber.

If your eating patterns are average, then your protein intake is about twice the amount required for body building and repair. The surplus is either burned as energy or stored as fat. In addition to being associated with fat, animal protein is also a more concentrated source of calories than vegetable protein. So cutting down on animal protein is a natural way to stay slim. It also helps to fortify you against some major problems: heart disease, cancer, high blood pressure, osteoporosis (softening of the bones), diverticular disease (an inflammation of the intestines) and kidney stones.

If you're eating more animal protein than you need, begin cutting down on your portions of meat, substituting potatoes, grains and vegetables. Combining vegetables with grains, legumes or low fat dairy products will enable you to design meatless meals with nourishing good taste which still provide you with a complete protein.

Fat: Energy, Insulation and Contouring

Fat is a highly concentrated source of energy. The fats in your food are carriers for certain vitamins and aid in the absorption of vitamin D from sunlight. Surplus protein and carbohydrates, as well as excess dietary fats, are converted by your liver into body fat for reserve energy. Deposits of fat surround, protect and hold in place your kidneys, liver, heart and other organs, while a layer of sub-surface fat helps you to preserve body heat, insulates you from environmental fluctuations, and rounds out the contours of your body. Fat is the primary source of slower burning fuel for body heat and muscular activity.

Fat consumption has been on the rise over the past hundred years, not only because of its presence in sources of animal protein, but also because of a wider availability and use of refined fats and oils, particularly margarines and salad oils. Fat is far and away the most concentrated source of calories, so high-fat meals are also high-calorie meals. Further, high-fat meals require more energy to digest, and may give you a sleepy, lethargic feeling. They may also produce heartburn.

While your body does need a variety of fats daily, you're likely to get most of what you need from your protein and carbohydrate sources without having to eat outright fats such as butter, margarine, mayonnaise, salad dressings and oils. In other words, what you eat of these items is essentially for taste and not for nourishment. So it's a good idea to keep your intake of fats to a minimum. Remove visible fat from the meats you eat. Take the skin off of turkey and chicken. And when you do use fats, watch the amount.

Other ways you can reduce your intake of fats are by using low fat, or better yet, skim dairy products, and by avoiding fried foods, including most "fast foods."

Salt

Processed foods tend to be high in salt, or sodium, in its many forms. They also tend to be low in the potassium ordinarily present in many unprocessed foods. Increased reliance on convenience foods has given rise to a sodium-potassium imbalance which is reflected in a growing incidence of high blood pressure, or hypertension. About one in five adults has high blood pressure, though only about half know it. Unattended, it can lead to arterial disease, heart attack, stroke or kidney failure. You can increase your intake of potassium by eating more fresh fruits, especially bananas, and fresh vegetables. Cut down on your use of salt in cooking and at the table. Use other herbs and spices for flavor.

Eat Well!

No doubt about it, there's a lot to be said for eating well, and the rewards are great. And remember, this is not a "don't" routine. Nor is it a "should" routine. This is simply eating intelligently, in a way that fits the realities of living well within a human body.

The payoffs can be relatively immediate: you'll notice an increase in your energy level, shinier hair, clearer skin and perhaps more sparkle in your eye. Common discomforts like constipation, heartburn and anemia will decrease or disappear. And over the long haul, your eating patterns will promote extraordinary health and well-being.

The basic principles of nutrition:

1. Regularly eat a well-balanced variety of fresh, unprocessed grains, fruits, vegetables and low-fat dairy products.
2. Eat little meat, and when you do, select those that are low in fat. Remove skin and any visible fats from your meats prior to preparation.
3. Minimize your intake of fats, sugar and salt.

TABLE OF FOOD COMPOSITION

Item	Meas-ure	Calo-ries	Grams Carbos.	Grams Pro-tein	Grams Fat	Grams Fiber
Beverages						
Beer	1 cup	101	9.1	.7	.0	
85 proof liquor	1 oz	70	.0	.0	.0	
Wine, sweet	1 cup	329	18.4	.2	.0	
Wine, dry	1 cup	204	9.6	.2	.0	
Coffee	1 cup	5	.8	.3	.0	
Tea	1 cup	4	.9	.1	.0	
Cola drinks	1 cup	94	19.0	.0	.0	
Fruit soft drinks	1 cup	110	29.0	.0	.0	
Dairy Products						
Cheddar cheese	1 oz	112	.4	7.0	9.4	
Colby cheese	1 oz	112	.7	6.7	9.1	
Cottage cheese-2%	1 cup	203	8.2	31.0	4.4	
Monterey jack	1 oz	106	.2	6.9	8.6	
Mozzarella-skim	1 oz	79	.9	7.8	4.9	
Parmesan, hard	1 oz	110	.8	10.0	7.3	
Egg, raw	1 lg	82	.5	6.5	6.4	
Egg white, raw	1 lg	17	.3	3.6		
Egg yolk, raw	1 lg	59	.1	2.8	5.7	
Condensed milk	1 cup	982	166.0	24.8	26.6	
Dried whole milk	1 cup	635	49.2	33.7	34.2	
Dried nonfat milk	1 cup	435	62.4	43.4	.9	
Skim milk	1 cup	86	11.8	8.4	.4	
Whole milk	1 cup	159	11.4	8.5	8.2	
Yogurt, whole milk	8 oz	139	10.6	7.9	7.4	
Yogurt, low-fat	8 oz	144	16.0	11.9	3.5	
Desserts & Sweets						
Brownies-2x2x¾"	1 pc	146	15.3	2.0	9.4	.2
Devils food cake, no icing-2x3x2"	1 pc	165	23.4	2.2	7.7	
Chocolate icing	1 cup	1034	185.0	8.8	38.2	
Chocolate milk bar	1 oz	147	16.1	2.2	9.2	
Choc. chip cookie	2½" dia.	51	6.0	.6	3.0	
Oatmeal cookie	3" dia.	63	10.3	.9	2.2	
Raised doughnut	1 plain	124	11.3	1.9	8.0	
Honey	1 tbsp	64	17.3	.1	.0	
Beet or cane sugar	1 tbsp	46	11.9	.0	.0	
Jams & preserves	1 tbsp	54	14.0	.1	.0	
Apple pie	1 pc	410	61.0	3.4	17.8	.6
Pecan pie	1 pc	668	82.0	8.2	36.6	.8
Fruits, Nuts & Juices						
Apple, raw	1 med	96	24.0	.3	1.0	.7
Apple juice, unsw	1 cup	117	29.5	.2	1.0	
Avocado, raw pitted	1 avg	334	12.6	4.2	32.8	3.2
Banana, raw	1 avg	127	33.3	1.6	.3	.8
Cantaloupe, raw	1 avg	30	7.5	.7	.1	.3
Dates, pitted	10 med	274	72.9	2.2	.5	2.3
Grapefruit, raw	½ med	41	10.8	.5	.1	.2
Orange, raw	1 avg	64	16.0	1.3	.3	.9
Orange juice, unsw	1 cup	112	25.8	1.7	.5	
Pineapple, raw	1 cup	81	21.2	.6	.3	.5
Pineapple juice	1 cup	138	33.8	1.0	.3	.2
Raisins, packed	1 cup	477	128.0	4.1	.3	1.4
Almonds, raw	1 cup	849	27.7	26.4	77.0	3.9
Peanuts, roasted	1 cup	838	29.7	37.7	70.1	3.9
Peanut butter	1 tbsp	86	3.2	3.9	8.1	.3
Coconut, fresh	1 cup	277	7.5	2.8	28.2	
Meat, Poultry & Seafood						
Chuck roast	1 lb.	905	.0	78.8	75.0	
Ground beef, lean	1 lb.	812	.0	93.9	45.4	
Ground beef, reg.	1 lb.	1216	.0	81.2	96.2	
Beef liver	1 lb.	140	5.3	19.9	17.3	
Chicken breast	1 lb.	394	.0	74.5	18.0	
Chicken thigh	1 lb.	435	.0	61.6	33.5	
Frankfurter	1 lb.	1402	8.2	56.7	131.0	
Pork chops	1 lb.	1065	.0	61.0	89.0	
Ham, cured	1 lb.	1535	1.2	66.7	138.0	
Bologna	1 lb.	1379	5.0	54.9	133.0	
Pork sausage	1 lb.	2259	.0	42.6	230.0	
Salami	1 lb.	2041	5.4	108.0	151.0	
Turkey, dark meat	1 lb.	921	.0	136.0	37.6	
Turkey, light meat	1 lb.	798	.0	149.0	17.7	
Bass	1 lb.	472	.0	85.7	9.5	
Flounder & sole	1 lb.	358	.0	75.8	5.4	
Halibut	1 lb.	454	.0	94.8	5.0	
Lobster	1 lb.	413	2.3	76.7	8.6	
Shrimp, fresh	1 lb.	413	6.8	82.1	3.6	
Tuna, canned in oil & drained	1 cup	315	.0	46.1	13.1	
Tuna, canned in water	1 cup	254	.0	56.0	1.6	
Dressings, Oils & Fats						
Mayonnaise	1 tbsp	101	.3	.2	11.2	
Blue or roquefort	1 tbsp	76	1.1	.7	7.8	
Italian	1 tbsp	83	1.0	.0	9.0	
Thousand island	1 tbsp	80	2.5	.1	8.0	
Soy sauce	1 tbsp	12	1.7	1.0	.2	
Butter	1 tbsp	102	.1	.1	11.5	
Margarine, regular	1 tbsp	102	.1	.1	11.5	
Margarine, whipped	1 tbsp	68	.0	.1	7.6	
Safflower oil	1 tbsp	124	.0	.0	14.0	
Soups						
Chicken noodle	1 cup	62	7.9	3.4	1.9	.3
Clam chowder- New England	1 cup	130	10.5	4.3	7.7	.3
Mushroom, cream of	1 cup	134	10.1	2.4	9.6	.1
Onion	1 cup	65	5.3	5.3	2.4	.5
Tomato	1 cup	88	15.7	2.0	2.5	.7
Vegetables, Legumes, Sprouts & Juices						
Alfalfa sprouts	1 cup	41		5.1	.6	1.7
Beans, canned	1 cup	300	57.6	15.8	1.2	3.6
Kidney beans	1 cup	230	41.8	14.5	1.0	2.3
Soybean curd (tofu)	3½ oz	72	2.4	7.8	4.2	.1
Broccoli, cooked	1 cup	40	7.0	4.8	.5	2.0
Brussels sprouts	1 cup	56	9.9	6.5	.6	
Cabbage, cooked	1 cup	29	6.2	1.6	.3	
Carrots, cooked	1 cup	48	11.0	1.4	.3	
Carrots, raw	1 lg	42	9.7	1.1	.2	1.0
Carrot juice	1 cup	96	22.2	2.5		
Cauliflower	1 cup	28	5.1	2.9	.3	
Celery, raw	1 cup	20	4.7	1.1	.1	.7
Corn, cooked	1 cup	137	31.0	5.3	1.7	
Corn, cream style	1 cup	210	51.2	5.4	1.5	
Eggplant, cooked	1 cup	38	8.2	2.0	.4	1.8
Lettuce, iceberg	1 cup	10	2.2	.7	.1	.4
Mushrooms, raw	1 cup	20	3.1	1.9	.2	
Onions, cooked	1 cup	61	13.7	2.5	.2	1.2
Peas, cooked	1 cup	114	19.4	8.6	.6	3.2
Potatoes, baked	1 lg	145	32.8	4.0	.2	1.2
French fries	10 pcs	137	18.0	2.1	6.6	.5
Potatoes, scalloped	1 cup	255	36.0	7.4	9.6	
Potato chips	10 chips	113	10.0	1.1	8.0	.3
Spinach, raw	1 cup	14	2.4	1.8	.2	.3
Squash, summer	1 cup	25	5.6	1.6	.2	.8
Tomato, raw	1 med	33	7.0	1.6	.3	.8
Tomato juice	1 cup	46	10.4	2.2	.2	.4
Veg. juice cocktail	1 cup	41	8.7	2.2	.2	.8
Yeast, bakers' dry	1 oz	80	11.0	10.5	.5	
Grains & Grain Products						
Pita, whole wheat	1 avg	140	24.0	6.0	2.0	
Bread, white enr.	1 slice	62	11.6	2.0	.8	
Bread, whole wheat	1 slice	56	11.0	2.4	.7	.4
Graham crackers	1 lg	55	10.4	1.1	1.3	.2
Soda crackers	1 avg	12	2.0	.4	.4	
Flour, wheat enr.	1 cup	400	83.7	11.6	1.1	.3
Flour, whole wheat	1 cup	400	83.7	11.6	1.1	2.8
Noodles, egg enr.	1 cup	200	37.3	6.6	2.4	.2
Oatmeal-rolled oats	1 cup	132	23.3	4.8	2.4	.5
Pancakes, plain enr.	4"diam	62	9.2	1.9	1.9	.1
Pancakes, whole wht	4"diam	74	8.8	3.4	3.2	
Pizza, cheese-14"	⅛	153	18.4	7.8	5.4	.2
Popcorn, plain	1 cup	54	10.7	1.8	.7	.3
Rice, white-cooked	1 cup	223	49.6	4.1	.4	.2
Rice, brown-cooked	1 cup	178	38.2	3.8	1.2	.5
Shredded wheat bskt	1 avg	89	20.0	2.5	.5	.5
Spaghetti, cooked	1 cup	155	32.2	4.8	.6	.2
Tortilla, corn	6"diam	63	13.5	1.5	.6	.3
Wheat germ, raw	1 cup	363	46.7	26.6	10.9	2.5
Wheat germ, toasted	1 cup	368	48.0	29.0	11.2	1.7

Blanks indicate that values have not been established.

Not surprisingly, proper weight is very much an individual matter. For example, a six foot football player might have a proper weight of 230 pounds, while a sprinter of the same age, sex and height might have a proper weight of 165 pounds. That's because what matters is not actually your weight, but the amount of fat you're carrying as compared to your productive body mass — your muscle, bone and organ tissue. In this country, as many as eight out of ten people carry more fat than is desired for optimal efficiency. A healthy ratio of body fat to total body mass ranges from 8 to 15 percent for adult males, and from 15 to 22 percent for females.

Maintaining a weight that is right for you is an important aspect of preserving your health for a lifetime. If you are of normal weight for a person your height, sex and body build, you are likely to live longer, have more energy and feel better than if your weight is above normal. Overweight is associated with many health problems, including atherosclerosis, heart disease, stroke, kidney trouble, diabetes, high blood pressure, malnutrition, inactivity and impaired self-image. It's clearly worth the effort to keep your weight under control.

Of course, for most people the question isn't whether or not it's worth the effort. What it usually boils down to is how to do it — reliably, safely and relatively painlessly so you can go on living as you like without losing your capacities along the way.

The first principle of an effective weight control program is to make sure that it is capable of working over the long haul. Crash weight loss programs are notorious for their failure rates because they are not nutritionally sound to begin with. Any weight that *is* lost, and often this is mostly water, tends to be quickly regained when the temporary program is discontinued and the old patterns are resumed. Effective weight control is an important strategic element of your general lifestyle, rather than a "quick-fix" reaction to your present condition.

Your body forms fat when the food you eat contains more calories, or energy value, than you are able to use at the time. On the other hand, when you expend more calories than you're taking in, some of your body fat is burned to make up the difference, thereby reducing your overall body weight. So you can lose weight by eating properly, by becoming more active, and, of course, by doing both at the same time.

Food bulk is not what produces fat. Surplus calories produce fat. By increasing your intake of fiber-rich fruits, vegetables, whole grains and legumes, while decreasing your intake of high calorie meats, sugars, fats and alcohol, you will have gone a long way toward gaining control of your weight. Ounce for ounce, carbohydrates contain only half the calories of fat, so replacing fats, fried foods and fatty meats with unrefined carbohydrates cuts your caloric intake considerably, without giving you the feeling that you're starving yourself in the process.

Activity

In addition to proper nutritional intake, weight control is a matter of energy expenditure — burning up the calories you're consuming in your food. When you are generally inactive, your body chemistry is altered so that fewer calories are burned as you perform all your normal daily activities. On the other hand, when you regularly engage in physical activity of some intensity, your muscles produce more of the chemicals that convert blood sugar and fat into energy. You're also signalling to your body that it needs strength and endurance to

Body composition. The proportion of your total body mass that is properly composed of fat depends upon your sex, body build and patterns of activity. Generally speaking, a healthful body composition for women is about 18 percent, and for men about 13 percent.

A few people, like male marathon runners, may get to as low as 5 percent; while Eskimo peoples, who live active lives in close contact with the arctic elements, may be in excellent physical condition yet carry a higher than average percentage of body fat as protective insulation.

Surplus fuel is stored in special fat cells located throughout your body. Every pound of excess fat requires an extra 200 miles of capillaries, taxing your entire cardio-respiratory system for its support.

The key factor in weight control is balancing the calories you're taking in with the calories you're expending in your daily activities.

meet the demands you're placing upon it, so more protein is diverted to the building of muscle and organ tissue. These changes persist in your body long after the period of activity itself, so that even while you are sitting at your desk or sleeping in bed, your body is burning more calories and preparing itself for the next exertion. This yields dividends in the form of more muscle and bone, less fat, more energy and improved concentration.

Understanding the process by which fat is produced is only a part of the solution. To gain lasting weight reduction requires altering any patterns of thought, feeling or behavior that may be contributing to your weight problem. If you have been overweight for some time, it's likely that you have adjusted your self image so that you now think of yourself as "being fat" — at least to some extent. And, when you think of yourself in this way, it's entirely consistent for you to feel and act as a "fat person" might.

One of the most important steps you can take — perhaps the easiest step — is to readjust your self image so that you think of yourself as a thin, trim, healthy and active person. Initially this is done through the use of your imagination. By seeing, feeling and accepting yourself as one who is naturally well-proportioned, you prepare the way for acting toward the realization of this result.

Your feelings or emotions are also a part of your behavioral patterning. Eating is sometimes used in an effort to satisfy other needs, such as the need for love, social acceptance or excitement. Or it may be used to relieve uncomfortable feelings like loneliness, boredom, tension, fear or depression. These feelings may then become associated with excessive or otherwise nutritionally unbalanced eating, often bringing effects which are exactly the opposite of those intended — more depression or loneliness etc.

Become aware of any self-defeating associations that may exist between your patterns of eating and your emotional state. Then identify things you can do which can be more realistically expected to resolve the difficulty. When you notice that you are experiencing the emotion, bring your thin self image to mind, and take whatever action you have determined to be more effective.

To help you develop a clear image of yourself as a thin person, remember yourself at another time when you may have been more trim. If you have any pictures of yourself as a thin person, get them out and look at them, visualize yourself now as you were then. Allow yourself to feel what you felt like at that time. You may want to put a picture up for you to see each day. If you have always been overweight, then find models for the way you want to look in magazines. When you see someone whose shape you admire, visualize yourself as having that shape. Never allow yourself to make unfavorable comparisons between yourself and anyone else, as this will tend to undo the work you have done on your new self image.

Set realistic goals for yourself, remembering that it took a long time for you to gain the extra weight you now have. Be patient with yourself. Shedding a pound or two each week is plenty. Over a year that adds up to between 50 and 100 pounds!

Some Weight Loss Tips

If you have some extra fat to lose, take advantage of any obvious opportunities you have for reducing your caloric intake. For example:

Put less food on your plate.
Stop eating **before** you feel full.
Leave some food on your plate.
Don't go back for seconds.
Remove your plate when you have finished.
Leave leftovers for another meal.
Pass up desserts, or have fresh fruit instead.
Cut down on your intake of alcohol.
Stay active — get daily exercise.
Don't starve yourself.
Don't rely upon diet pills.
Avoid greasy fast foods.
Shop for groceries when you're full.
Don't eat while doing other things.
Avoid snacks between meals — especially sweets.
Select the foods you eat with care for yourself.
Remember to eat veggies.
Avoid double applications of fats — butter and salad dressing or sour cream and cheese.
Avoid fruit "drinks."

What Is Stress?

Your body responds, sometimes dramatically, to each of your emotions. Its natural response to fear is to mobilize for efficient defensive action with the so-called **"fight-or-flight" response**. At the extreme, this is what happens:

- once your brain is activated, it calls for release of chemicals into the bloodstream which signal an emergency to the rest of your body;

- your chest expands to draw more oxygen into your lungs;

- your heart and blood vessels dilate, and your blood pressure rises to accelerate the flow of vital fluids throughout your body;

- your liver releases glucose into the bloodstream to fuel your muscles;

- your muscles contract in preparation for immediate movement;

- your skin surface blood vessels contract, causing your skin to pale;

- your blood coagulates quickly if your skin is punctured;

- your pupils dilate and your eyelids open to maximize your vision;

- perspiration increases, goose bumps form and your hair stands on end to improve body cooling;

- your bladder and intestines may empty themselves of unnecessary matter.

This is the incredible response which allows a 100 pound woman to lift a 3,000 pound automobile from her child.

Marvelous as it is, this response can do great damage to your body when it is not given adequate release. Yet hard running and physical defense are seldom called for in dealing with the typical challenges of modern living, such as job pressures, financial uncertainties, family and social obligations, and more generalized cultural concerns like environmental deterioration and the nuclear threat. Chronic, low grade stimulation of your powerful fight-or-flight response has detrimental effects on your body's regulatory, nervous, circulatory and immunological systems.

Clearly this is an area deserving of your closest attention. Fortunately, stress is not an inherent quality of your external circumstances. It is a response to your circumstances which takes place inside of you, and is therefore subject to your personal control. This is evident from the great differences observable among individual responses to the same set of circumstances.

Goal Clarity and Personal Organization

Stress management begins with setting your own directions by establishing worthwhile goals for yourself. Your goals need to be **realistic** in the sense that they effectively address the actual circumstances of your life. At the same time, they need to be **idealistic** in the sense that they properly reflect your noblest intent, and encompass your highest aspirations. Make it a point to insist that each of your goals incorporates this harmonious blend of practical realism and genuinely rewarding idealism. Though at times this may require the expenditure of some creative energy, you'll gradually discover that it's never necessary to settle for anything less.

You're more likely to realize your goals when they are stated in terms that are

The early effects of chronic unrelieved stress may include headaches, stomach upsets, sleeplessness, hypertension, lower back pain, psychosomatic illnesses, anxiety, irritability, mental disorientation smoking, alcohol and drug abuse.

Longer term effects may include heart disease, stroke, cancer, ulcers, narrowing and hardening of the arteries, obesity and alcoholism. The extent of the problem is reflected in the fact that valium, which temporarily masks some of the symptoms of acute distress, is one of the most prescribed drugs in the world today.

Stress management amounts to taking control of yourself. Not in an impatient, critical and punitive sense, but in a caring, compassionate, yet firmly determined sense. Stress management means taking good care of yourself, and appreciating yourself for who you are. Not because you've earned it, but because you are, by your nature, deserving of respect and appreciation. From this central point of strength, you can extend your attitude of peace, acceptance, appreciation, confidence and determination, first to others, and then to the entire world of your personal experience.

simple, clear and specific. **The more clearly you specify your true choice in any situation, the more likely this favorable outcome becomes.** It's only common sense, yet all too easily forgotten when your attention is captivated by your circumstances, as so often happens when you are "under stress."

To develop a clear image of your goals for yourself, use as many of your faculties as possible. For example, in addition to **seeing** the realization of your goals, you gain even greater clarity and certainty by **feeling** what it's like for them to be fulfilled, and by **accepting** them as already accomplished within the realm of your creative consciousness.

In carrying out these goal clarification exercises, everything you visualize is seen in the present, and the language you use in describing your goals to yourself is also stated in the present, rather than in the future. In this way you give yourself a more complete experience of what it's like to have already accomplished the task that you have set for yourself. This enables you to further specify your goal, and prepares you for the experience of realizing it.

Begin your goal clarification exercise by relaxing yourself in a comfortable position where you will not be disturbed. Close your eyes and then see, feel and accept yourself as already **being** the person you choose to be. Visualize yourself in as much detail as possible, relating honorably and effectively to the realities of your current life situation. Use your imagination and enjoy yourself. Next see and feel yourself **doing** what you choose to do, again in as much detail as possible. Then see and feel what it's like to **enjoy having** the things that come with being and doing as you have chosen.

This exercise creates a well-rounded picture of your goal in very specific, concrete and personal terms. It specifies your inner state of being — your identity, as well as your behavior and your outer environment — what you have.

In accomplishing these exercises, don't allow any negative self-talk to enter in. At this point you are not attempting to figure out how you are going to achieve your goal. You are simply identifying what the goal is. This is a good way to eliminate any negative, self-defeating assumptions that you may have been laboring under.

When you experience yourself as already being the person you choose to be, your behavior tends to become consistent with this new self-image. In this way you're not fighting yourself for a change in behavior. Instead, the desired behavior flows naturally from your newly adopted self-concept.

Clarity and personal organization are the necessary underpinnings for effective functioning on a moment-by-moment basis in the course of your daily affairs. Check yourself regularly to assure that you are enjoying a clear sense of who you are and where you're headed with respect to all the important areas of your life. There's no need to live with nagging dissatisfactions and chronic feelings of helplessness when you can far more easily turn your experience around with a bit of determination and creative problem solving.

Attitude Control

Stress is associated with specific attitudes and behaviors. These include: impatience, inability to relax without feeling guilty, excessive competitiveness, aggressiveness, inability to listen attentively without thinking of other things, strong motivation toward obtaining external rewards and recognition, an immoderate need for information and control, a pervasive sense of personal responsibility, and a highly judgmental attitude.

In order for your goals to be practically useful to you in the present, they must be stated in concrete terms that are responsive to your immediate circumstances, and respectful of your true potential as an individual.

Stress places you in a reactive relationship to your circumstances, while effective stress management puts you in control of yourself with respect to your circumstances.

On the positive side, there's a set of corresponding attitudes and behaviors which are not only highly effective, but also conducive to lasting good health. For example, the much admired ability to remain calm, self-possessed and efficient in a tight situation. Or the ability to listen attentively and empathetically to others when they are speaking. There's also being supportive of others and rejoicing in their successes, rather than indulging in jealous competition. Or being able to humbly acknowledge your true feelings and to discuss those matters that are of greatest importance to you. Others include thoroughly enjoying the experience of living and being human, quite apart from the gratifications of external rewards and recognition; and appreciating yourself and others for having performed at your personal peak, aside from any comparative results which may come from your actions.

Your goal clarification activities are ideally suited for installing these and other positive attributes as characteristic traits of your personality. In addition, you can exercise attitude control to handle those cases in which your observed response to a situation is inconsistent with your preferences. For example, you may choose to be a patient, tolerant person, yet observe that in certain circumstances you become impatient and highly critical. Your natural response upon making such an observation might be to turn your impatience and criticism back in upon yourself, thereby even further complicating matters.

When you find yourself in the midst of an undesirable reaction, you're in need of a means of consciously diverting your energy and attention along the lines of your true preferences. Fortunately, at this point you have already taken the first, most crucial step in exercising control over your attitude — you have noticed what you are doing. It is important that you not attempt to directly oppose what you are doing, since this is likely to prolong and complicate your reaction. Instead, provide yourself with a suitable alternative to the course you are on.

Begin by quickly establishing an adequate perspective. Acknowledge the relationship between the momentary events at hand and the full sweep of your life — from your birth to your eventual death. This can be accomplished in an instant, and has the beneficial effect of shrinking the illusion of importance that events so readily acquire when they are viewed solely within a narrow temporal context.

The next step is the most delicate: begin focusing all of your attention on the specific elements of the situation, without allowing yourself to pass judgment on any aspect of what is taking place. Occupy your attention with pure, concentrated observation, noticing exactly what is happening as an interested observer, without drawing conclusions, and without attempting to justify, explain or criticize anything whatsoever.

From this position of detached observation, you are far more likely to become aware of all the options available to you in relating to the situation at hand, including your preferred ways of thinking, feeling and behaving. And here's where your preparatory goal clarification work really pays off. In many cases, a tasteful touch of good humor may be all that's needed to immediately transform the entire situation from tense to relaxed. The key point is that you are acting in accordance with your conscious choice, rather than remaining bound within an unpleasant chain of unrewarding reactions.

Obstacles to successful attitude control are habitual patterns of negative self-talk. Your attitudes are shaped by what you say to yourself in your on-going mental conversation. The private "movies" you play for yourself while driving home from work or while taking a shower fortify your position within the world of your experience. Begin watching this flow of imagery from a stress management point of view, inserting the kinds of suggestions you'd like to see yourself living out. Learn to expect the best — from yourself, from others, and from the world in general. Anxiety gives way to enthusiasm with increasing mastery of life.

Conscious Relaxation

The physiological responses associated with stress and anxiety are incompatible with deep muscle relaxation. This means that by fully relaxing your entire body, and along with it your mind and emotions, you can break the hold of chronic stress, diminishing its influence upon your body and your life. Interestingly, conscious relaxation has stress reducing effects that cannot be provided by simply sitting quietly or even by sleeping. Your body waits to be told that it's safe to relax; otherwise, it may faithfully hold itself in a state of perpetual readiness, regardless of what you may be doing.

The regular practice of conscious relaxation also develops the essential skills which underlie both powerful personal goal-setting, and reliable attitude control. To do either with full effectiveness requires cultivation of your ability to interrupt and divert — at will — the automatic flow of imagery which otherwise passes uninterruptedly across the field of your consciousness. Taking positive control of your life implies a growing facility for channeling your thoughts, and thereby your emotions and actions, in the directions that you choose for yourself when you are at your very best.

Conscious relaxation is a simple process in which first your body, and then your mind and emotions, are gradually brought to a point of silence — a tranquil state which is then purposefully maintained for a short period of time. At the end of this quiet period, you are ideally situated for your goal clarification activity, free of any conflicting thoughts, feelings or sensations. As you become more adept in the practice of quieting your mind, your capacity for making instantaneous adjustments in your attitude will also grow.

This conscious relaxation procedure is adapted from extensive research conducted by Herbert Benson, M.D., and first reported in his best-selling book "The Relaxation Response." It is an effective method of releasing yourself from the grip of chronic tension.

1. Select a place where you will not be disturbed. Sit quietly in a comfortable position with your eyes closed.

2. Deeply relax all your muscles by placing your attention upon them one at a time, beginning with the muscles of your feet and working all the way up to the muscles of your face. Allow your body to remain relaxed.

3. Breathe through your nose. Become aware of your breathing, and as you breathe out, say a single word or phrase silently to yourself. This phrase can be neutral in meaning, such as the word "one," or it can be any other expression which has a calming and empowering effect upon you. Continue observing your breathing, while repeating your chosen word or phrase to yourself with each exhalation. Do this for at least five minutes at the outset, gradually lengthening your period of conscious relaxation to as long as twenty minutes. You may open your eyes to check the time, but do not use an alarm. After you finish, sit quietly for a few minutes, at first with your eyes closed, then with them open. If you are planning a goal clarification exercise, do it at this time, prior to opening your eyes.

Don't worry about whether you are successful in achieving a "deep level of relaxation". Just maintain a receptive attitude and permit relaxation to occur at its own pace. Expect other thoughts, and allow them to pass undisturbed when they occur. Simply breathe them out with a quiet "one." With practice, full relaxation will come to you without effort.

Regular exercise burns off excess energy and removes any free-floating chemicals that may be left over from "emergencies" you have encountered in the course of your day. Regular aerobic activity tends to reduce depression, lower your blood pressure and heart rate, improve the quality of your sleep, and strengthen your self-esteem. And the extra strength, energy and body efficiency you gain from exercising helps to prepare you for the mental, physical and emotional challenges you encounter.

A dependency may arise from the regular use of any drug taken for the purpose of altering your mood. The drugs most commonly used for mood alteration are tobacco, caffeine, alcohol and sedatives, amphetamines, marijuana, cocaine, narcotics and hallucinogens.

Each of these substances has physical effects in addition to its psychoactive, or mind-altering properties. Most of them can seriously damage your body when taken in large amounts or over an extended period of time.

With repeated use, the body also develops a tolerance for certain drugs, requiring larger or more frequent doses for the same mood-altering effect.

Tobacco: Cigarette smoking is considered by many authorities to be the largest single preventable cause of illness and premature death in this country. Tobacco is associated with an estimated 320,000 premature deaths a year, and another 10 million people currently suffer from debilitating chronic diseases caused by smoking. It is associated with heart and blood vessel diseases; chronic bronchitis and emphysema; a number of cancers, especially cancer of the lung; and stomach ulcers. Smoking also increases the risk of complications of pregnancy and retardation of fetal growth.

Alcohol: Misuse of alcohol is a factor in about 200,000 deaths a year. It is associated with half of all traffic deaths, many involving teenagers. Cirrhosis, one of the ten leading causes of death, is largely attributable to alcohol. Alcohol use is also associated with cancers of the liver, esophagus and mouth. While even moderate drinking is a risk during pregnancy, excessive drinking may lead to severe infant abnormalities. Ten million adults are estimated to be alcoholics or problem drinkers. On the average, heavy drinkers shorten their life span by about 10 years.

Sedatives: Sedatives are misused by at least one million Americans, and 30,000 are estimated to be addicted to them. Barbiturate withdrawal is often more severe than heroin withdrawal, with abrupt withdrawal sometimes leading to convulsions which may produce permanent disability or even death. Overdosing with barbiturates is a leading cause of drug overdose fatalities. Combinations of barbiturates with depressants, particularly alcohol, are extremely risky.

Caffeine: Caffeine, which stimulates the central nervous system, can produce anxiety, gastritis, heartburn and sleeplessness.

Marijuana: Marijuana is currently used by an estimated 16 million persons. Over time, smoking five marijuana cigarettes a week is as damaging to the lungs as smoking about six packs of cigarettes a week. Marijuana use affects hormonal balance, including both sex and growth hormones. It may reduce fertility in women and sperm count in men. Marijuana may be especially harmful during adolescence — a period of rapid physical and sexual development. Marijuana may also have a toxic effect on embryos and fetuses. THC, the psychoactive ingredient in marijuana, is measurable in urine up to ten weeks after usage, and even longer in blood samples. This means that frequent usage has a cumulative effect — increasingly destabilizing the body chemistry. This may be reflected in loss of sex drive, exaggerated mood swings and a general feeling of lethargy. Many of these effects appear to quickly recede after usage is discontinued.

Physical and Psychological Dependence

Regular use of any mood altering substance produces at least some degree of psychological dependence — that is, a reliance upon it to make you feel good. Certain of the substances also produce a physical dependence because of adjustments the body makes to accommodate them. After these adjustments have been made, the body becomes distressed when it is deprived of the drug. The most physically addictive substances are barbiturates, alcohol, cocaine, narcotics and tobacco. Others which appear to be physically addictive, though to a lesser extent, are amphetamines, caffeine and marijuana.

By now you're probably asking yourself: "How can I put all this valuable information to work in my life?" The Positive Lifestyling program provides you with an efficient and enjoyable means of systematically building these desirable patterns of living into your accustomed way of life. Positive Lifestyling is a pleasant wellness game that you can begin playing right now, and continue to enjoy for the rest of your life . . . for just as long as you like. The benefits to you never stop rolling in.

You'll note that, for the most part, Positive Lifestyling focuses your attention on adding desirable new behaviors to your present way of life, rather than on changing or eliminating old behaviors. This new complex of healthful activities has the welcome effect of gradually easing out many of the less desirable patterns without raising even the hint of a struggle.

Positive Lifestyling is a cyclical program, with each cycle lasting six weeks. At the beginning of each six-week period, complete the Lifestyle Inventory, taking a full reading on your present status across all the key wellness categories. You've probably completed this step for your first cycle already. With this overview to work from, you're then prepared to select a set of Positive Lifestyling goals for yourself to accomplish during the upcoming six weeks. These goals are chosen from among 13 wellness-related categories covering the areas of stress management, physical activity, nutrition and chemical independence. Weight control is a product of five of these 13 categories.

Having selected your goals, stay with them — unchanged — for the following 42 day period. At the beginning of each week, record your weight and resting heart rate in the progress charts provided. You'll be able to monitor and record your daily performance using the convenient Positive Lifestyling log forms which are provided. Keep track of your activity in all areas. At the end of each week, tally up your performance scores and translate them into colors for entry on your Long-Term Progress Record.

Upon completion of the six-week cycle, you'll once again be ready to retake your Lifestyle Inventory. This provides you with a comprehensive picture of how you're doing with respect to the full array of wellness-related lifestyle factors, and prepares the way for you to establish new wellness goals for the next cycle.

In setting your goals, remember not to overdo it. At first you may be attracted by the idea of taking on all of the behaviors described in the workbook at once. Obviously there's nothing wrong with this, and you can certainly accomplish it if you set your mind to it. In fact, you'll no doubt discover that you're making more healthful choices on a daily basis in a number of areas where you haven't even set goals as of yet. Just bear in mind that the most important ingredient of effective Positive Lifestyling is your eventual success with it. It's far more desirable for you to gradually achieve mastery in all or most areas over a period of a year or two than it is for you to give up in needless frustration after a few weeks of trying to take on more than you may be ready for at the moment.

For the greatest measure of success, you may prefer to select just a few key factors to focus on at any one point. These would be aspects of your lifestyle that you really feel ready to polish up at that time. When you've identified one, two, or perhaps three such items, that may be plenty for the moment. In any case, don't overload yourself with an array of things that you think you "should"

Positive Lifestyling provides you with 13 wellness-related objectives from which you may select your current set of personal wellness goals:

In the area of Stress Management:
- Conscious Relaxation
- Goal Clarity and Personal Organization
- Attitude Control

In the area of Physical Activity:
- Full-Body Stretching
- Cardio-Respiratory Activity
- Body Toning

In the area of Nutrition:
- Eating Independence
- Unrefined Carbohydrate Intake
- Fat Intake

In the area of Chemical Independence:
- Caffeine Intake
- Alcohol Intake
- Drug Intake
- Tobacco Use

Weight management is accomplished through five of the thirteen Positive Lifestyling objectives:
- Conscious Relaxation
- Cardio-Respiratory Activity
- Eating Independence
- Unrefined Carbohydrate Intake
- Fat Intake

Live out your plan of action for the next six weeks. Make that commitment to yourself at the outset. Approach it as a six week experiment in taking charge of your life. Don't be bothered by any initial resistances you may feel — just accept them as a matter of course, and keep right on going.

So get yourself started right now — today. There's no better way for you to invest your time and attention. The payoffs are enormous, and they keep right on coming in, day after day, year after year for the rest of your life.

be doing, without assuring that you do, in actual fact, feel ready to carry them out. Use your goal clarification exercises to bring yourself to this point.

Over the long term, you'll find that persistence and determination are your most valuable Positive Lifestyling assets. When you're not entirely satisfied with your progress, simply reaffirm your determination and continue to persist in the healthful course that you have chosen for yourself. Reinforce your new self-image — your personal wellness goal — every day with at least a few minutes of quiet, relaxed visualization, perhaps while driving your car or before dropping off to sleep at night. Then renew it again when you awaken in the morning. Do this until you become so familiar with this new image of yourself that any other ideas feel foreign to you. Don't allow yourself to indulge in any contrary visions of who you are becoming. When they do occur, simply substitute your image of the new you in their place.

And remember to reward yourself for your accomplishments. The changes you're making have great long-term value, and immediate rewards recognize and reinforce your success right now.

Always bear in mind that your life is entirely yours to live, and that you deserve the best, regardless of anything you may have experienced up to now. At first you may feel a little like you're swimming upstream — you and everyone else who knows you expect you to think, feel and act according to your familiar patterns. But soon you'll notice that you're becoming more comfortable acting in ways that are consistent with your new self-concept, and that your old patterns are beginning to feel like last year's wardrobe — a little out of fashion. Let them go! Before you know it, you'll be completing your first six-week cycle, and you'll be successfully launched on a new, healthier way of living — **choosing your way** to lasting health and well-being.

PLANNING CALENDAR

This Positive Lifestyling Planning Calendar is provided to assist you in the scheduling of your conscious relaxation and physical activity sessions. You may also find it useful in gaining an overview of the way you are utilizing your time in general.

Begin by taking a look at how your time is now allocated. If you sleep 8 hours a day, and you work 40 hours per week, then you have about 72 hours each week to use in other ways. Your weekly calendar might look something like this:

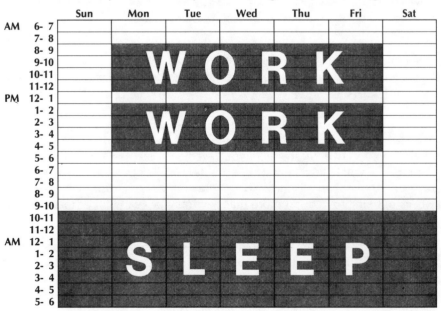

To create your own personalized calendar, first color in the blocks representing the days and hours that you customarily spend at work, using one color of pencil or crayon. Next, using a different color, fill in the blocks that represent your usual hours of sleep. You may want to use a third color to identify any other times that are already committed to regular weekly activities, such as classes you might be attending. As you proceed through the various sections which follow, you'll be able to note the times for your various Positive Lifestyling activities in the remaining spaces of your calendar.

		Sun	Mon	Tue	Wed	Thu	Fri	Sat
AM	6- 7							
	7- 8							
	8- 9							
	9-10							
	10-11							
	11-12							
PM	12- 1							
	1- 2							
	2- 3							
	3- 4							
	4- 5							
	5- 6							
	6- 7							
	7- 8							
	8- 9							
	9-10							
	10-11							
	11-12							
AM	12- 1							
	1- 2							
	2- 3							
	3- 4							
	4- 5							
	5- 6							

STRESS MANAGEMENT

Positive Lifestyling begins with stress management because the powerful stress response influences virtually every aspect of your experience:

- Your awareness of who you are and of your true intent;
- Your focus of attention;
- Your feelings, sensations and perceptions;
- Your emotions, intuitions, interpretations and judgments;
- Your recollections of past experiences;
- Your envisioned and expected future experiences;
- Your attitude toward yourself and your world;
- Your expression in word, in gesture, and in deed.

Harmonizing these fundamental forces and putting them to constructive work in your life is what stress management is really all about. You can break the hold of chronic stress in your life with these three Positive Lifestyling strategies:
    first, regularly practice conscious relaxation;
    second, maintain your clarity and personal organization; and
    third; exercise positive attitude control.

Conscious Relaxation

The physiological responses associated with stress and anxiety are incompatible with deep muscle relaxation. When you fully relax yourself once or twice each day, you open the door to taking positive control over every other aspect of your life. For this reason, conscious relaxation is an essential first step in the successful practice of Positive Lifestyling. If you are not already accustomed to engaging in some form of conscious relaxation, begin now by setting a specific time for it each day, allowing at least 10 minutes per session at the outset. Pick a convenient time, considering your current schedule, and then enter these periods onto your activity calendar with a letter "C" in the appropriate blocks for each day of the week.

Clarity and Personal Organization

Stress management involves determining your own directions by setting worth-while goals for yourself. The more clearly you are able to specify your true preferences with respect to the key circumstances of your life, the more likely you are to experience their ultimate fulfillment. Clarity and personal organization are the product of a continuous process, involving the sorting out of confusions, the reduction of uncertainty and doubt, and the constructive rechanneling of such emotions as fear, anger, hatred, envy or guilt.

After you have completed your period of conscious relaxation, and while you are still in a relaxed, receptive frame of mind, take a few minutes to **vividly see, feel and accept yourself** as already being precisely the person you most truly choose to be, handling every situation in ways that are entirely consistent with your chosen self, and enjoying all the benefits that come from being and doing your very best.

Accustom yourself to performing this clarifying and organizing activity regularly, so that you are always possessed of a relatively unconflicted image of yourself in connection with every important aspect of your life. When you notice that you're unclear about something, enter into your conscious relaxation period with a confident awareness that you are patiently awaiting the emergence of clarity in the troubled area. Then, upon completion of your conscious relaxation exercise, begin mentally describing yourself in complete detail, just as you most truly choose to be. Don't allow yourself to indulge in any negative thoughts or emotions, no matter how enticing they may seem. When they do occur, simply replace them with their positive counterparts.

At times this may call for a degree of concentration and determination, but you'll soon discover that it is infinitely easier than attempting to sort out confusions, unguided, within the shifting context of onrushing daily experience.

Attitude Control

With your self-image and direction clearly established, the next step is to make sure that you're staying on track in the course of your daily affairs. Having already privately experienced your preferences with respect to all the key situations in your life, you're well prepared to enjoy the rewarding experience of living them out.

Attitude control is your moment by moment choice of orientation with respect to the ever-shifting circumstances of life. At each point in time, you may either act in accordance with your conscious choice, or fall back upon prior habit patterns. Ordinarily the choice is easy, and your prior visualizations place you in the perfect position to smoothly realize your preferences.

However, when a perceived threat arises, it may trigger the physiologically compelling "flight-or-fight" response, which in turn tends to throw your entire system into a more or less automatic reaction. Under these conditions, your spontaneous thought and behavior will tend to reflect the patterns which you habitually associate with the feelings which prevail at that time. It is at precisely these moments that your awareness of who you are can be called to your aid. Recognize yourself as the author of your life, take a deep breath, relax your body, quiet your mind, still your emotions, and insert your preferred self-image directly into the flow of experience. Restore your full capacity for noble and effective action.

Three types of physical activity are recommended within the Positive Lifestyling program: full-body stretching, cardio-respiratory activity, and body toning. Each of these makes a distinct contribution to your level of wellness.

Full-body stretching

In addition to maintaining the flexibility and range of motion of your major muscles and joints, stretching is a necessary preliminary to safely performing both aerobic and body toning activities. So if you're planning to begin with just one of the three types of recommended activity, then daily full-body stretching is a natural way to get started.

Choose a convenient time for your daily stretch — perhaps upon arising in the morning or in the quiet of the evening, or just prior to any aerobic or body toning workouts you have planned. Performing the 13 recommended Positive Lifestyling stretches for 15 to 30 seconds each takes just ten minutes a day. Enter these periods into your schedule with a letter "S" in the appropriate blocks for each day.

Cardio-respiratory activity

When you're ready to participate in two of the three types of recommended activities, add a complete five-part cardio-respiratory workout to your daily full-body stretches. Engaging in an aerobic workout once each day is ideal, while every other day is adequate. By performing your full-body stretches just prior to your aerobic activity, they can serve as the first part of your aerobic workout — the pre-exercise stretch.

Select aerobic activities that you'll enjoy, such as swimming, bicycling, jogging, walking, rowing, dancercise or basketball. It's not necessary that the activity be the same each day. For example, you may enjoy playing a game of racquetball two or three times a week. While this is an excellent form of physical activity, it may not provide you with a complete aerobic workout in your target training range. However, when performed in combination with a more aerobic activity — such as swimming — on the off-days, the two can work together to keep you in great shape with a high level of enjoyment.

After you have decided which aerobic activities you'd like to perform, determine where and when you are going to accomplish them. Be specific, considering how to fit them into your schedule, and allowing sufficient time for travel and a shower afterwards. To complete all five parts of your aerobic workout, set aside at least 25 minutes at the outset, gradually building up to 45 minutes or more per session. Enter your aerobic periods into your schedule with a letter "A" in the appropriate blocks. Make sure that you obtain any necessary equipment well in advance of your first scheduled session.

Whatever you do, **don't allow yourself to overdo it.** This is a common tendency during the first few times out, when you may be inclined to expect your performance to be at the same level as you may have experienced years ago. To get a realistic idea of how to proceed, review the easy progressions outlined in the walking and jogging programs provided on page 19. Once again, patient

Cardio-respiratory activity is one of the five elements of the weight management complex. If you are 25 percent or more overweight, your weight-loss objective will be most readily achieved through frequent bouts of extended aerobic activity, perhaps undertaken initially at the low end of your target training range, so that you can sustain them for longer periods. This has the effect of burning off more calories initially, while preparing you for the more vigorous activity that you'll be performing as your conditioning improves. Walking, bicycling, swimming and rowing are excellent activities for the overweight person, with the latter three placing minimal stress on the hips, knees, ankles and feet.

determination and persistence are your greatest Positive Lifestyling assets, while impatience and procrastination are ever-threatening thieves of the success that you deserve, and that you can surely achieve.

Body toning

When your stretching and aerobic programs are firmly in place, you're ready to begin your body toning activity. Body toning is effective when performed two or three times each week in addition to your daily stretching and aerobic activities. Precede your body toning workouts with full-body stretches and follow them up with the brief set of post-exercise stretches. You can tone all of your major muscles — thighs (front & back), calves, stomach, waist, chest, shoulders, back and arms — in just 15 to 20 minutes per session. Enter your body toning periods into your schedule with a letter "T" in the appropriate blocks.

Certain body toning exercises can be performed with sufficient vigor and regularity to maintain your heart rate in its target training range. For example, some slimnastics classes are conducted in this way. If this is the case with the body toning activity that **you** prefer — and you can check this by noting your pulse rate during the workout — then your body toning exercises can also satisfy your aerobic requirements on the days when you perform them.

NUTRITION

Positive Lifestyling provides you with three nutritional objectives: optimal intake of unrefined carbohydrates, moderate intake of fats, and eating independence. Each of these is an important contributing factor in the five-part weight management complex.

Optimizing your intake of unrefined carbohydrates:

Step 1. If fresh fruit is not already a regular part of your daily food regimen, concentrate during the first week on adding fruit to your eating patterns. First shop for some good looking fruit — bananas, apples, oranges, grapefruit, peaches, melons, grapes etc. — and then make sure that you have at least one serving of it each day. Fruit makes an excellent snack, and may be effectively substituted for sweets to help you break the sugar habit.

Step 2. Add fresh raw vegetables daily. While continuing to eat fresh fruit each day, this week add some fresh raw vegetables to your daily food intake. Shop for greens like lettuce, spinach, romaine, parsley, watercress or mint. Also try such things as carrots, celery, cucumbers, green peppers, cabbage, cauliflower, and tomatoes. Treat yourself to an attractive, tasty fresh salad each day. And try carrots or celery as a snack in place of sweets.

Step 3. Add fresh steamed vegetables. While continuing with your fruit and fresh raw vegetables on a daily basis, this week add fresh (or frozen) steamed vegetables to at least one meal each day. Shop for some broccoli, green beans, peas, corn, carrots, brussel sprouts, cauliflower, cabbage or asparagus — whatever seems good to you. It's better to lightly steam your vegetables than to cook them in water, since this helps to keep the good flavor and nutrients inside.

Step 4. Continue taking raw and steamed vegetables and fresh fruit each day while adding a daily serving of whole grains. Shop for grain products that are not highly processed and that contain as little sugar and preservatives as possible. These products might include breads, dry and cooked cereals, tortillas, rolls or muffins. Even cakes and pie crusts can be made using whole wheat and honey. Try substituting noodles and macaroni made from vegetables and whole grains for those made from highly processed wheat. Use brown rice rather than white. Among the cereals, there are many, both cooked and uncooked, which taste great and contain little or no added sugar or preservatives. Try a variety of grains, including wheat, oats, rice, corn, barley, rye and bulgar or cracked wheat.

Moderating your intake of fats.

Step 1. Low fat protein. This week make it a point to add protein from low fat sources to your daily food intake. Shop for meats like turkey, chicken and fish instead of high-fat meats such as pork, prime beef, hamburger, duck and lamb. Include high protein vegetables like dried beans, lentils and split peas. Remove the skin from turkey and chicken during preparation. Ground turkey is generally available if you ask your butcher shop for it, and it serves as an excellent substitute for hamburger in virtually all applications.

Step 2. Add low-fat or non-fat dairy products. Continue with your intake of low-fat meats, this week adding low-fat or non-fat dairy products in place of whole milk and other full-fat dairy products. Margarine is better than butter; soft margarine is better than hard margarine. Also cut down on your use of fats like butter, margarine, oils and salad dressings, and minimize your intake of deep fried foods.

CHEMICAL INDEPENDENCE

If your use of any chemical substance is detracting from your general state of well-being, begin now to reestablish a more rewarding balance. In the discussion which follows, the example of smoking is used to illustrate the procedures, but the same approach can be applied to the elimination of any potential dependency.

Step 1. Clearly determine for yourself that you are entitled to live your life independent of any potentially damaging chemical substances; that you are entirely capable of granting yourself this independence; and that you are unwilling to settle for anything less than enjoying the full measure of physical health, emotional balance and psychological freedom that is your birthright.

It is in the nature of dependencies that they present the illusion of holding power over the will of the individual. If you're like most people, you aren't entirely comfortable with the idea that anything has power over your will to act in your own best interests. Yet many people are reluctant to challenge an ingrained habit for fear that there may be a high price to pay in terms of physical discomfort and mental distraction. In short, they are held hostage by the threat of losing the temporary sense of well-being which they have become accustomed to giving themselves through the use of the chemical. Eventually their inherent capacity for the experience of joy itself may be compromised by the gradual transfer of this great personal power from themselves to an external object — a chemical substance.

If you have grown accustomed to using one or more chemical substances — caffeine, alcohol, tobacco or other drugs — take the first step now. Consciously claim your right to stay well and to live free of any encumbering dependencies. For now, do this without concern for how you will accomplish it, and without anticipating any difficulty or discomfort. Simply establish this as a necessary principle for healthful, joyous living, which somehow or other you are determined to implement within your life.

Step 2. Closely observe and record your use of any chemical substance that has the potential of becoming a dependency. Observe without exercising judgment or attempting to intervene in any way. Notice as many details as possible — the circumstances, your feelings and thought patterns, your moods, your words and your behavior. And remember, do nothing but watch and keep a record at this time . . . without even a judgment. Simply pay close attention to all the dynamics of your use of the substance as an interested, yet completely detached observer. Give no thought to the idea of altering your patterns, other than to keep a record of your usage, including the amount, the time, the circumstances, the effects — both immediate and subsequent — and any other observations you may make. If you find that you're resisting this step, simply take note of that fact, along with everything else, and continue to observe and record whatever is taking place.

Step 3. Adopt the point of view that you are freeing yourself of any dependency that may be threatening you at this time. Approach it as an experiment in positive self-control and effective decision-making. This means knowing from the outset that you are not interested in engaging in any struggle or in tolerating any nagging discomforts. What you are determined to accomplish is the feat of actually becoming, with the totality of yourself, a person who is truly a non-smoker, a non-drinker or whatever.

To illustrate, you wouldn't want to approach smoking cessation as a smoker who is trying to quit. Such an approach is virtually guaranteed to engage you in a knock-down, drag-out fight with yourself, because while continuing to see yourself as one who smokes — a smoker, you're demanding of yourself the elimination of the very behavior that goes along with being a smoker — smoking. Instead of engaging in this type of internal conflict, adopt the more effective strategy of actually becoming a non-smoker first. In this way you can simply live out the thoughts, feelings and behaviors that flow naturally from the enjoyment of this essential state of well-being.

Some typical suggestions to give yourself when becoming a non-smoker might be: "I am a completely healthy person who consistently acts in ways that promote my greatest well-being. I enjoy breathing clean, fresh air into my lungs. My lungs are clear and full of life, providing smoke-free oxygen to my entire body. My hands are clean and odor free, as are my clothes, my home and my car. The air in my home, my place of work and my automobile is fresh and life-giving. I enjoy eating and drinking in moderation in a clean-smelling, smoke-free environment. I am completely unaffected by the smoking practices of other people, and am indifferent to what they do with tobacco. I arise in the morning to the pleasant smell of fresh air, and look forward to another invigorating day of living and breathing well . . . ."

Amazing though it may seem, you can readily accomplish this through the determined use of your creative imagination in your goal clarification exercises. And, as you know, the more comprehensive and realistic you are able to make the image of yourself as a non-smoker, the easier it is for you to live it out in your daily life. The experience of millions of people has shown that by using this approach, it is entirely possible for you to thoroughly reprogram yourself as a non-smoker one evening before going to bed, and then to awaken in the morning as a non-smoker who never again feels even the slightest inclination to touch a cigarette.

When you have completed the development of your self-image as a non-smoker, give yourself a few instructions for handling the situations that are likely to come up. For example, when you awaken in the morning, be prepared to carry on as a non-smoker, without paying any attention to it, unless something should arise which raises the issue of smoking. If a friend who thinks of you as a smoker offers you a cigarette, or if something else occurs which brings up the question as to whether or not you would like to smoke, be prepared to immediately ask yourself one simple question: "Am I a smoker; or am I a non-smoker?" Do this before you have had an opportunity to think of anything else, or to engage in any deliberations that might otherwise be triggered by the offer of a cigarette. And then be prepared to accept whatever answer you get back without a struggle.

If the answer you receive is that you are a smoker, then you know that your reprogramming activity is not complete. If the answer is that you are a non-smoker, then there is no problem, and the situation calls for no further attention or thought. Accept yourself as a non-smoker and continue to carry on as though nothing could be more natural. Don't make anything special out of it.

When someone asks you if you have quit smoking, respond by acknowledging that you aren't smoking. Don't allow yourself to become involved in anyone else's idea of how difficult it is to "quit." Until you have accumulated some time as a non-smoker, it's probably best not to talk about what you are doing, and not even to think about it yourself. Simply allow yourself to be what you have chosen to become.

On the other hand, if you should discover that you are still a smoker, then return once again to the creative process of goal clarification, with the patient determination that you are, in fact, becoming a non-smoker, non-drinker etc., and that it is simply a matter of time until this result is fully realized in your life. You may supplement your personal work with professional assistance if that appears to be needed.

Alcohol

Alcoholism is now recognized as a severe illness which manifests itself both physically and behaviorally. In most areas, qualified professional assistance is readily available to treat this illness during its acute stages, and to provide valuable follow-through services.

In a culture where alcohol is commonly used as a social lubricant, the probability of repeated exposure to alcohol is high. For the majority of people, light consumption of alcohol appears to be relatively safe. Yet for many others this is not the case. The ingestion of alcohol is ill-advised during pregnancy, in combination with certain medications, or when recovering from some illnesses.

Alcohol is also unsafe, even in small doses, for a large and diverse population of people who seem to possess a physical predisposition to alcohol addiction. That is, when they engage in the practice of drinking, they're more likely than others to drink to excess, and to eventually fall prey to a dependency. These people appear to have a higher than average tolerance of the initial mood altering effects of alcohol. That is, when drinking moderate amounts of alcohol, they experience a less intense mood-altering effect than do most other people. Yet beyond a certain threshold point, they become just as intoxicated as anyone else who has consumed a like amount. It's a biologically predetermined all-or-nothing setup which carries with it a higher susceptibility to the formation of a major chemical dependency.

At this time, there is no reliable way of testing for this predisposition beforehand. Consequently millions of people discover the problem only after they have already fallen victim to it. If you are one of these, take advantage of the best available assistance now. And remember to treat yourself to a refreshing new self-image as a non-drinker.

Conclusion.

Allow the enormous wisdom and power of the being that grows your body, heals your wounds and regulates your overall functioning to be expressed through you, and to bring about a full healing of every aspect of yourself that needs it. Let the process work in the same way that you allow yourself to breathe, to sleep, to dream and to remember. Give yourself regular access to the full scope of your personal capacity for achieving wholeness, and for enjoying wellness for life.

HOW TO USE THE DAILY PERFORMANCE RECORD

Perhaps the single most effective step that you can take at this moment to expand your share of wellness is to begin monitoring your lifestyle patterns in the thirteen key areas discussed throughout the workbook. By continuing to systematically monitor your actual behavior, you'll assure yourself of gradually building an ever increasing measure of well-being into your life. Here are a few additional comments which may assist you in completing the Daily Performance Record.

Clarity and Personal Organization

Staying on track in all the important areas of life is aided by focusing on specific aspects at different times. Each week, give yourself the assignment of paying particular attention to your degree of clarity and personal organization in one major area. Here is a suggested cycle:

Week 1 — Relationships with family and friends.
Week 2 — Recreational activities and directions; community service.
Week 3 — Relationships with co-workers, associates and acquaintances.
Week 4 — Occupational activities, aspirations, directions and goals.
Week 5 — Financial patterns, aspirations and goals.
Week 6 — Environmental quality in your home, at work, in your community.

Attitude Control

Effective attitude control can also be aided by focusing on a variety of desirable attributes, one at a time. Each day, pay particular attention to the quality of your internal state with respect to one attitudinal factor. Add new factors to keep this list fully responsive to your own personal needs.

Day 1 — Openness, friendliness, attentiveness to others.
Day 2 — Honesty, forthrightness, expressiveness.
Day 3 — Playfulness, spontaneity, enjoyment of life.
Day 4 — Humor, sense of perspective, appreciation of incongruities.

Day 5 — Forgiveness.
Day 6 — Appreciation of self and others.
Day 7 — Confidence.
Day 8 — Positive recollections of past events.
Day 9 — Positive anticipations of future events.
Day 10 — Patience, tolerance of delays and imperfections.
Day 11 — Determination.
Day 12 — Assistance to others, supportiveness, cooperation.
Day 13 — Concentration.
Day 14 — Caring for others, compassionate understanding.

Amount of Food Eaten

Moderate eating involves eating less than would be required to fill your stomach at meals, and not eating substantial amounts between meals. If you're overweight, chances are your stomach is stretched and out of tone. By never filling your stomach, you give it an opportunity to recover its normal healthy shape and tone. This also permits the most efficient digestive action to take place. In general, if you are eating good nutritious foods, and you're still gaining excessive weight, then you are consuming more food than your activity level warrants.

Intake of Unrefined Carbohydrates

Fresh fruit, fresh raw vegetables, fresh or frozen steamed vegetables, and whole grains are the foods which qualify as unrefined carbohydrates. To obtain all the energy and nutrients you need to feel good, stay strong, and perform well, your total daily food intake should consist primarily of these readily digested foods.

Intake of Fats

The major sources of fats are meats — especially red meats, full fat dairy products, deep-fried foods, and fat derivatives such as butter, margarine, mayonnaise, salad dressings and oils. A moderate intake of fats would consist of little meat, low-fat or non-fat dairy products, and minimal fat derivatives.

Place a mark in the "Goal" column of the Daily Performance Record to designate those objectives which you have selected as personal goals for this six-week cycle.

Keep a daily record of your performance by filling in the appropriate dot for each objective.

At the end of each week, summarize your performance.
- First, count the number of dots in each line and enter the totals in the "#" column.
- Next, multiply these totals by the number given in the "X" column, and enter this product in the " = " column.
- Add up the two or three products associated with each objective, and enter the results in the "Total" column.
- Use these totals to arrive at your Weekly Weight Management and Positive Lifestyling Indices.
- Transfer all of your Weekly totals to the Long-Term Progress Record provided on pages 57.

DAILY PERFORMANCE RECORD – WEEKS 1 & 2

	GOAL	OBJECTIVE		Week 1 S M T W T F S	#	X	=	Total	Week 2 S M T W T F S	#	X	=	Total
STRESS MANAGEMENT	A	Clarity and Personal Organization	clear & organized	o o o o o o o		45			o o o o o o o		45		
			a bit disorganized	o o o o o o o		30			o o o o o o o		30		
			poorly organized	o o o o o o o		15			o o o o o o o		15		
	B	Attitude Control	positive attitude	o o o o o o o		90			o o o o o o o		90		
			mostly positive	o o o o o o o		60			o o o o o o o		60		
			negative attitude	o o o o o o o		30			o o o o o o o		30		
	C	Conscious Relaxation	at least 5 minutes	o o o o o o o		75			o o o o o o o		75		
			less than 5 minutes	o o o o o o o		25			o o o o o o o		25		
PHYSICAL ACTIVITY	D	Full-Body Stretching	stretched	o o o o o o o		60			o o o o o o o		60		
			didn't stretch	o o o o o o o		20			o o o o o o o		20		
	E	Most Recent Aerobic Workout	this day	o o o o o o o		120			o o o o o o o		120		
			the day before	o o o o o o o		80			o o o o o o o		80		
			2 or more days prior	o o o o o o o		40			o o o o o o o		40		
	F	Most Recent Body Toning Workout	this day	o o o o o o o		30			o o o o o o o		30		
			1 or 2 days before	o o o o o o o		20			o o o o o o o		20		
			3 or more days prior	o o o o o o o		10			o o o o o o o		10		
NUTRITIONAL INTAKE	G	Amount of Food Eaten	moderate	o o o o o o o		60			o o o o o o o		60		
			a bit too much	o o o o o o o		40			o o o o o o o		40		
			excessive	o o o o o o o		20			o o o o o o o		20		
	H	Intake of Unrefined Carbohydrates	high	o o o o o o o		75			o o o o o o o		75		
			medium	o o o o o o o		50			o o o o o o o		50		
			low	o o o o o o o		25			o o o o o o o		25		
	I	Intake of Fats	low fat	o o o o o o o		75			o o o o o o o		75		
			medium fat	o o o o o o o		50			o o o o o o o		50		
			high fat	o o o o o o o		25			o o o o o o o		25		
CHEMICAL INDEPENDENCE	J	Caffeine	1 cup or less	o o o o o o o		0			o o o o o o o		0		
			2-3 cups	o o o o o o o		-5			o o o o o o o		-5		
			more than 3 cups	o o o o o o o		-10			o o o o o o o		-10		
	K	Alcohol	1 serving or less	o o o o o o o		0			o o o o o o o		0		
			2 servings	o o o o o o o		-10			o o o o o o o		-10		
			3 or more servings	o o o o o o o		-40			o o o o o o o		-40		
	L	Drugs	minimum possible	o o o o o o o		0			o o o o o o o		0		
			more than minimum	o o o o o o o		-40			o o o o o o o		-40		
	M	Tobacco	didn't smoke	o o o o o o o		0			o o o o o o o		0		
			smoked	o o o o o o o		-50			o o o o o o o		-50		

Weekly Weight Management Index
(sum of items C + E + G + H + I)

Weekly Positive Lifestyling Index
(sum of all items)

Keep a daily record of your performance by filling in the appropriate dots — See instructions on page 50.

DAILY PERFORMANCE RECORD — WEEKS 3 & 4

	GOAL	OBJECTIVE		Week 3 SMTWTFS	#	X	=	Total	Week 4 SMTWTFS	#	X	=	Total
STRESS MANAGEMENT	A	Clarity and Personal Organization	clear & organized	o o o o o o o		45			o o o o o o o		45		
			a bit disorganized	o o o o o o o		30			o o o o o o o		30		
			poorly organized	o o o o o o o		15			o o o o o o o		15		
	B	Attitude Control	positive attitude	o o o o o o o		90			o o o o o o o		90		
			mostly positive	o o o o o o o		60			o o o o o o o		60		
			negative attitude	o o o o o o o		30			o o o o o o o		30		
	C	Conscious Relaxation	at least 5 minutes	o o o o o o o		75			o o o o o o o		75		
			less than 5 minutes	o o o o o o o		25			o o o o o o o		25		
PHYSICAL ACTIVITY	D	Full-Body Stretching	stretched	o o o o o o o		60			o o o o o o o		60		
			didn't stretch	o o o o o o o		20			o o o o o o o		20		
	E	Most Recent Aerobic Workout	this day	o o o o o o o		120			o o o o o o o		120		
			the day before	o o o o o o o		80			o o o o o o o		80		
			2 or more days prior	o o o o o o o		40			o o o o o o o		40		
	F	Most Recent Body Toning Workout	this day	o o o o o o o		30			o o o o o o o		30		
			1 or 2 days before	o o o o o o o		20			o o o o o o o		20		
			3 or more days prior	o o o o o o o		10			o o o o o o o		10		
NUTRITIONAL INTAKE	G	Amount of Food Eaten	moderate	o o o o o o o		60			o o o o o o o		60		
			a bit too much	o o o o o o o		40			o o o o o o o		40		
			excessive	o o o o o o o		20			o o o o o o o		20		
	H	Intake of Unrefined Carbohydrates	high	o o o o o o o		75			o o o o o o o		75		
			medium	o o o o o o o		50			o o o o o o o		50		
			low	o o o o o o o		25			o o o o o o o		25		
	I	Intake of Fats	low fat	o o o o o o o		75			o o o o o o o		75		
			medium fat	o o o o o o o		50			o o o o o o o		50		
			high fat	o o o o o o o		25			o o o o o o o		25		
CHEMICAL INDEPENDENCE	J	Caffeine	1 cup or less	o o o o o o o		0			o o o o o o o		0		
			2-3 cups	o o o o o o o		-5			o o o o o o o		-5		
			more than 3 cups	o o o o o o o		-10			o o o o o o o		-10		
	K	Alcohol	1 serving or less	o o o o o o o		0			o o o o o o o		0		
			2 servings	o o o o o o o		-10			o o o o o o o		-10		
			3 or more servings	o o o o o o o		-40			o o o o o o o		-40		
	L	Drugs	minimum possible	o o o o o o o		0			o o o o o o o		0		
			more than minimum	o o o o o o o		-40			o o o o o o o		-40		
	M	Tobacco	didn't smoke	o o o o o o o		0			o o o o o o o		0		
			smoked	o o o o o o o		-50			o o o o o o o		-50		

Weekly Weight Management Index
(sum of items C + E + G + H + I)

Weekly Positive Lifestyling Index
(sum of all items)

To assure that you don't run out of Daily Performance Record forms, place your order now using the convenient order form provided.

DAILY PERFORMANCE RECORD – WEEKS 5 & 6

	GOAL	OBJECTIVE		Week 5 SMTWTFS	#	X	=	Total	Week 6 SMTWTFS	#	X	=	Total
STRESS MANAGEMENT	A	Clarity and Personal Organization	clear & organized	o o o o o o o		45			o o o o o o o		45		
			a bit disorganized	o o o o o o o		30			o o o o o o o		30		
			poorly organized	o o o o o o o		15			o o o o o o o		15		
	B	Attitude Control	positive attitude	o o o o o o o		90			o o o o o o o		90		
			mostly positive	o o o o o o o		60			o o o o o o o		60		
			negative attitude	o o o o o o o		30			o o o o o o o		30		
	C	Conscious Relaxation	at least 5 minutes	o o o o o o o		75			o o o o o o o		75		
			less than 5 minutes	o o o o o o o		25			o o o o o o o		25		
PHYSICAL ACTIVITY	D	Full-Body Stretching	stretched	o o o o o o o		60			o o o o o o o		60		
			didn't stretch	o o o o o o o		20			o o o o o o o		20		
	E	Most Recent Aerobic Workout	this day	o o o o o o o		120			o o o o o o o		120		
			the day before	o o o o o o o		80			o o o o o o o		80		
			2 or more days prior	o o o o o o o		40			o o o o o o o		40		
	F	Most Recent Body Toning Workout	this day	o o o o o o o		30			o o o o o o o		30		
			1 or 2 days before	o o o o o o o		20			o o o o o o o		20		
			3 or more days prior	o o o o o o o		10			o o o o o o o		10		
NUTRITIONAL INTAKE	G	Amount of Food Eaten	moderate	o o o o o o o		60			o o o o o o o		60		
			a bit too much	o o o o o o o		40			o o o o o o o		40		
			excessive	o o o o o o o		20			o o o o o o o		20		
	H	Intake of Unrefined Carbohydrates	high	o o o o o o o		75			o o o o o o o		75		
			medium	o o o o o o o		50			o o o o o o o		50		
			low	o o o o o o o		25			o o o o o o o		25		
	I	Intake of Fats	low fat	o o o o o o o		75			o o o o o o o		75		
			medium fat	o o o o o o o		50			o o o o o o o		50		
			high fat	o o o o o o o		25			o o o o o o o		25		
CHEMICAL INDEPENDENCE	J	Caffeine	1 cup or less	o o o o o o o		0			o o o o o o o		0		
			2-3 cups	o o o o o o o		-5			o o o o o o o		-5		
			more than 3 cups	o o o o o o o		-10			o o o o o o o		-10		
	K	Alcohol	1 serving or less	o o o o o o o		0			o o o o o o o		0		
			2 servings	o o o o o o o		-10			o o o o o o o		-10		
			3 or more servings	o o o o o o o		-40			o o o o o o o		-40		
	L	Drugs	minimum possible	o o o o o o o		0			o o o o o o o		0		
			more than minimum	o o o o o o o		-40			o o o o o o o		-40		
	M	Tobacco	didn't smoke	o o o o o o o		0			o o o o o o o		0		
			smoked	o o o o o o o		-50			o o o o o o o		-50		

Weekly Weight Management Index
(sum of items C + E + G + H + I)

Weekly Positive Lifestyling Index
(sum of all items)

After you have completed this six-week cycle, retake the Lifestyle Inventory, and establish your goals for the next six weeks

WEIGHT CONTROL PROGRESS CHART

CHART THE POUNDS WHICH YOU ARE LOSING EACH WEEK

WEEK	DATE	WGT	1	2	3	4	5	6	7	8	9	10	11	12	13	14	15	16	17	18	19	20	21	22	23	24	25
1																											
2																											
3																											
4																											
5																											
6																											
7																											
8																											
9																											
10																											
11																											
12																											
13																											
14																											
15																											
16																											
17																											
18																											
19																											
20																											
21																											
22																											
23																											
24																											
25																											
26																											
27																											
28																											
29																											
30																											
31																											
32																											
33																											
34																											
35																											
36																											
37																											
38																											
39																											
40																											
41																											
42																											
43																											
44																											
45																											
46																											
47																											
48																											

RESTING HEART RATE PROGRESS CHART

CHART THE REDUCTIONS IN YOUR RESTING HEART RATE EACH WEEK

WEEK	DATE	RATE	1	2	3	4	5	6	7	8	9	10	11	12	13	14	15	16	17	18	19	20	21	22	23	24	25
1																											
2																											
3																											
4																											
5																											
6																											
7																											
8																											
9																											
10																											
11																											
12																											
13																											
14																											
15																											
16																											
17																											
18																											
19																											
20																											
21																											
22																											
23																											
24																											
25																											
26																											
27																											
28																											
29																											
30																											
31																											
32																											
33																											
34																											
35																											
36																											
37																											
38																											
39																											
40																											
41																											
42																											
43																											
44																											
45																											
46																											
47																											
48																											

THE QUALITIES OF WELLNESS

MORE WELL		LESS WELL
Strengthened, circulates more blood per beat, permits lower resting heart rate.	Your Heart	Weakened, circulates less blood per beat, requires higher resting heart rate.
Larger, more elastic, less obstructed with fat, freer circulation, lower blood pressure.	Your Blood Vessels	Constricted, inelastic, clogged with excess fat, reduced circulation, elevated blood pressure.
Decreased cholesterol (fat), triglycerides, blood sugar, insulin, adrenalin, clotting.	Your Blood	Increased cholesterol (fat), triglycerides, blood sugar, insulin, adrenalin, clotting.
Expanded capacity for oxygen absorption and waste expulsion.	Your Lungs	Restricted capacity for oxygen absorption and waste expulsion.
Generally elevated, more calories consumed in all activities, promotes leanness.	Your Metabolic Rate	Generally suppressed, fewer calories consumed per activity, tends to accumulate more fat.
Lean, with proportionally more muscle and bone.	Your Body Composition	Fat, with proportionally less muscle and bone.
Stronger, more dense and resilient.	Your Bones	Weaker, more porous and brittle.
Capable of a wide range of fluid motion.	Your Joints	Stiff, restricted, sometimes painful motion.
Stronger, more firm, defined and efficient, tending to burn more calories.	Your Muscles	Weaker, less toned and efficient, tending to burn fewer calories, less sensitive to insulin.
Alert, more clear and concentrated, less boredom and fatigue.	Your Mental Functioning	Dull, worried and distracted, more boredom and fatigue.
More patient, tolerant, relaxed and enthusiastic.	Your Emotions	Impatient, critical, tense and depressed.
Decreased risk due to healthier heart, lungs, blood vessels, liver, bones, muscle and body composition.	Your Risk of Illness	Increased risk of diseases of heart, lungs, blood vessels and liver; of diabetes, stroke, accidents and broken bones.
More active, generating greater vitality and endurance, tending toward health.	Your Quality Of Life	Inactive, generating less vitality and endurance, tending toward illness.
Possible extension beyond the average.	Your Lifespan	Possible reduction below the average.
More confident, with positive appreciation of self.	Your Self-Concept	Less certain, more doubtful and self-conscious.

Enjoy the many lasting benefits of living a life of health, fitness and well-being.

LONG-TERM PROGRESS RECORD

Instructions: The Long-Term Progress Record provides you with a colorful display which enables you to see at a glance where your current living patterns are solidly supportive of your lasting well-being, and where they could use a bit of positive reinforcement. It also allows you to quickly recognize the progress you're making in the establishment of a well-balanced personal lifestyle for yourself.

To maintain this record, you'll need three different brightly colored pencils — red, yellow and green are ideal because of the powerful symbolic value which they already possess. Keep your Positive Lifestyle pens handy for ease of use whenever you need them.

At the end of each week, translate the Daily Performance Record weekly totals into their appropriate colors for entry here. Do this by referring to the "Mid-Range or Yellow Values" listed for each objective. When your weekly scores fall within these ranges, color the corresponding oval spaces yellow. When your scores are above the yellow range, color the ovals green. And when they fall below the yellow range, color those ovals red.

That's all there is to it. Simply update this visual record each week, and you'll always be in the perfect position to see exactly how you're doing across the entire array of key wellness factors. And best of all, it only takes a few moments for you to keep it up.

	Mid-Range or Yellow Values	CYCLE 1	CYCLE 2	CYCLE 3	CYCLE 4
	Wk	1 2 3 4 5 6	1 2 3 4 5 6	1 2 3 4 5 6	1 2 3 4 5 6
A. Goal Clarity	180-240				
B. Attitude Control	360-480				
C. Conscious Relaxation	275-375				
D. Stretching	220-300				
E. Aerobic Activity	480-600				
F. Body Toning	110-150				
G. Eating Independence	240-320				
H. Complex Carbohydrate	300-400				
I. Fat Intake	300-400				
J. Caffeine Independence	(35)-(15)				
K. Alcohol Independence	(40)-(20)				
L. Drug Independence	(40)				
M. Tobacco Independence	*				
Weight Management Index	1,535-2,135				
Positive Lifestyling Index	2,390-3,360				

* "0" equals green; any other score equals red.

BIBLIOGRAPHY

Exercise

Adult Physical Fitness, U.S. Government Printing Office, Washington, D.C. 20402.

Beyond Diet: Exercise Your Way To Fitness and Heart Health, Lenore Zohman. Pamphlet, free from Mazola Nutrition Information Service; Dept. ZD-NYT, Box 307, Conventry, Conn. 06238.

Exercise And Your Heart, Consumer Information Center, Box 3D, Pueblo, CO 81009. #555K.

Exercise in the Office, Robert R. Spackman (Carbondale, Ill.: Southern Illinois University Press, 1968).

Fit or Fat, Covert Bailey (Houghton Muffin Publishing Co., 1977).

How Mother's And Others Stay Slim, Lawrence Holt (California Health Publications, 1981).

Introduction to Yoga, Richard Hittleman (New York: Bantam, 1969).

Royal Canadian Air Force Exercise Plans For Physical Fitness (New York: Pocket Books, 1972).

Running For Health and Beauty: A Complete Guide For Women, Kathryn Lance (New York: Bobbs-Merrill, 1977).

The Complete Book of Running, James F. Fixx (New York: Random House, 1977).

The Miracle of Rebound Exercise, Albert E. Carter (Snohomish Publishing Co., Inc., 1979).

The New Aerobics, Kenneth Cooper (New York: Evans & Co., 1970).

The Perfect Exercise, Curtis Mitchell (New York: Simon & Schuster, 1976).

Booklets From The President's Council on Physical Fitness

These booklets can be purchased from: The Superintendent of Documents, U.S. Government Printing Office, Washington, D.C. 20402.

Adult Physical Fitness, S/N 040-000-00026-7.
Aqua Dynamics, S/N 040-000-00360-6.
The Fitness Challenge, S/N 017--62-00009-3.
Exercise and Weight Control, S/N 040-000-00371-1.
Youth Physical Fitness, S/N 040-000-00400-9.
One Step At A Time, S/N 017-001-00425-1.

Nutrition

Diet for a Small Planet, Frances Moore Lappé (New York: Ballantine Books, 1971).

The Eater's Guide, Candy Cumming and Vicky Newman (Spectrum Books, Prentice-Hall, Inc., 1981).

Let's Eat Right to Keep Fit, Adelle Davis (New York: Harcourt Brace Jovanovich, 1954).

Live Longer Now, Leonard, Hofer, and Pritikin (New York: Grosset & Dunlap, 1977).

Nutrition Almanac, Nutrition Search, Inc., John D. Kirschmann, Director (McGraw-Hill Book Company, 1979).

Orthomolecular Psychiatry, Linus Pauling (available from the Huxley Institute, 1114 First Ave., New York, N.Y. 10021).

Psychodietetics: Food as the Key to Emotional Health, Cheraskin, Ringsdorf, and Brecher (New York: Stein & Day, 1974).

Sugar Blues, William Dufty (New York: Warner, 1976).

Stress Management

Executive Health, Philip Goldberg (McGraw-Hill Publications, 1978).

Happiness, Bloomfield and Kory (New York: Simon & Schuster, 1976).

Management of Stress: Using TM at Work, David R. Frew (Chicago: Nelson-Hall, 1977).

Managing Stress: Before It Manages You, Steinmetz, Blankenship, Brown, Hall, and Miller (Bull Publishing Company, 1980).

New Mind, New Body, Barbara Brown (New York: Harper & Row, 1974).

Progressive Relaxation, Edmond Jacobson (Chicago: University of Chicago Press, 1938).

Relax, White and Fadiman, eds. (New York: Confucian Press, 1976).

Stress Without Distress, Hans Selye (Lippincott, 1974).

The Massage Book, George Downing (New York: Random House, 1972).

The Psychology of Consciousness, Robert Ornstein (San Francisco: W.H. Freeman & Co., 1972).

The Relaxation Response, Herbert Benson, (New York: Morrow, 1975).

The TM Program: The Way to Fulfillment, Philip Goldberg (New York: Holt, Rinehart & Winston, 1976).

TM and Business, Jay B. Marcus (New York: McGraw-Hill, 1978).

You Must Relax, Edmond Jacobson (New York: McGraw-Hill, 1957).

Dependencies

Clearing The Air, Consumer Information Center, Box 3D, Pueblo, CO 81009. #540K.

The following booklets and pamphlets can be purchased from: Alcohol, Drug Abuse & Mental Health Administration, 5600 Fishers Lane, Rockville, Maryland 20857.

Alcohol Abuse and Women, DHHS Publication No. (ADM) 80-358.

Drinking Etiquette, DHHS Pub. No. (ADM) 80-305.

Drug Abuse Prevention, DHHS Pub. No. (ADM) 81-584.

Let's Talk About Drug Abuse, DHHS Pub. No. (ADM) 80-706.

Someone Close Drinks Too Much, DHEW Pub. No. (ADM) 80-23.

The Drinking Question, DHHS Pub. No. (ADM) 80-286.

WELLNESS MATERIALS

Now You Can Experience POSITIVE LIFESTYLING On Your Own Personal Computer!

If you're lucky enough to have access to an IBM PC, XT or AT, then you're in for the healthful kick of a lifetime! Enjoy the colorful, graphically exciting and easily operated POSITIVE LIFESTYLING software program.

You'll be thoroughly entertained as the POSITIVE LIFE-STYLING program serves up the entire WELLNESS FOR LIFE system in a friendly, pleasantly interactive, menu-driven format. It's all here in dynamic graphics:

- The Lifestyle Inventory
- Comprehensive Wellness Library
- Cyclical Personalized Goal Setting
- Daily Performance Review
- Five-Point Weight Management Program
- Motivating Displays of Short & Long-Term Progress

You can comfortably share the POSITIVE LIFESTYLING program with your co-workers at the office, or with your entire family at home. It accommodates up to ten different users, each with private password protection to maintain the confidentiality of sensitive personal data.

And there's no problem if you travel frequently or have only periodic access to a computer. The POSITIVE LIFESTYLING software program is completely complementary to The WELLNESS FOR LIFE Workbook. Whenever necessary, you can use the workbook to maintain your daily records, then update your software files at the next convenient opportunity.

Order your copy of the exciting new POSITIVE LIFESTYLING software program today! Or, if you'd like a preview, send for our Demonstration Disk.

Requires IBM PC/XT/AT with dual disk drive, graphics adaptor and color monitor.

48-Week WELLNESS FOR LIFE Continuation Packet

Don't allow your supply of Positive Lifestyling materials to run out.

Order now the additional personal record-keeping forms you need to follow through on the valuable Positive Lifestyling program you've established for yourself. The handy 48-Week WELLNESS FOR LIFE Continuation Packet provides you with everything needed to complete eight 6-week Positive Lifestyling cycles — Lifestyle Inventories, Daily Performance Records, and Long-Term Progress Records. And the packet comes in two parts, so it can conveniently serve two people for 24 weeks each.

Send for your Continuation Packet today.

The WELLNESS FOR LIFE Workbook

Order additional copies of
The
WELLNESS FOR LIFE
Workbook
for your family, friends and co-workers.
There's no more thoughtful gift than
WELLNESS FOR LIFE.

Send to: Fitness Publications, P.O. Box 178554, San Diego, CA 92117

ORDER FORM

Enclosed is my check or money order for:

☐ _____ copies of The WELLNESS FOR LIFE Workbook at $6.95 plus $1.50 each for postage and handling.

☐ _____ 48-Week WELLNESS FOR LIFE Continuation Packets at $4.95 plus $1.50 each for postage and handling.

☐ _____ copies of the POSITIVE LIFESTYLING software program at $145 plus $5.00 each for postage and handling.

☐ A POSITIVE LIFESTYLING Demonstration Disk for $10 (postage and handling is included). I understand that this amount will be credited to the purchase price if I should decide to order the complete POSITIVE LIFESTYLING software program.

Where did you originally obtain your copy of The WELLNESS FOR LIFE Workbook? _____

How long have you been using the WELLNESS FOR LIFE system?

_____

Name_____

Address _____

City_____State_____Zip_____

ORDER FORM

Enclosed is my check or money order for:

☐ _____ copies of The WELLNESS FOR LIFE Workbook at $6.95 plus $1.50 each for postage and handling.

☐ _____ 48-Week WELLNESS FOR LIFE Continuation Packets at $4.95 plus $1.50 each for postage and handling.

☐ _____ copies of the POSITIVE LIFESTYLING software program at $145 plus $5.00 each for postage and handling.

☐ A POSITIVE LIFESTYLING Demonstration Disk for $10 (postage and handling is included). I understand that this amount will be credited to the purchase price if I should decide to order the complete POSITIVE LIFESTYLING software program.

Where did you originally obtain your copy of The WELLNESS FOR LIFE Workbook? _____

How long have you been using the WELLNESS FOR LIFE system?

_____

Name_____

Address _____

City_____State_____Zip_____